IN SEARCH OF THE PERFECT CLEANSE

by

Sir Jason Winters

VINTON PUBLISHING
P.O. Box 94075
Las Vegas, Nevada 89197

First edition – May, 1984
Twenty-sixth printing – May, 2006

ISBN – 1-885026-15-3
Library of Congress Catalog Card number pending.

Notice

I have reprinted this book exactly as my father wrote it over 23 years ago.

No part of this book is intended to replace any advice from your doctor. Please check with your doctor and/or health care practitioner if you are ill. The subject matter contained in this book is provided simply as information. In order that you may make your own informed decision after gathering as much information as you see fit. Please do not start on any diet, regimen, workout routine, or cleanse, that is contained in this book, unless you check with your doctor.

The author wishes to make it clear that he does not recommend total rejection of orthodox methods of treatment – or a doctor's advice. If you are ill see your doctor.

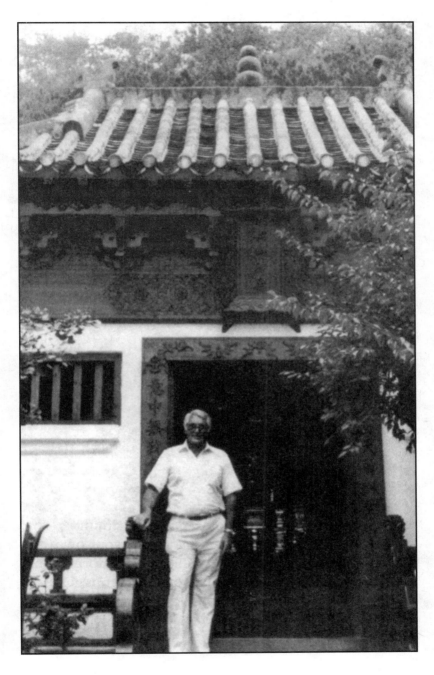

Jason Winters leaving the "Temple of Everlasting Happiness: in China.

...to turn around, but to face ... ...
the operating room. He was ...
...

Introduction:
CLEANSE

I seemed to be whirling through a large tunnel, with a great light at the end, yet I could still hear the voices of the doctors and nurses as they rushed around the operating room.

They I emerged from the tunnel into a brilliant, beautiful countryside, dazzling to the eyes. I was walking up a kind of embankment and below me on both sides were heavy dark mists so that I could not see the bottom. A great light was coming towards me and I could not step aside for it to pass because I would have then fallen into the darkness below.

The light passed through me and suddenly I was forced to turn around, only to find myself coming to in the operating room. The nurse said, "HE"S COMING AROUND, MORE ANESTHETIC," and I was back in the tunnel again.

I woke up in the hospital ward wrapped in bandages, only to be told by the doctor that I had terminal cancer with only weeks to live. That was over seven years ago. Since that time I have travelled the world, appeared on radio shows in almost every state and country to talk about one thing, and that is the cleansing of the body. By that I mean the mind, the skin, the nervous system, the cells and the colon, as well as the blood.

As you read through this book, you will find that we discuss the perfect way to cleanse each part of the body. One chapter will be devoted to the colon, said by many experts to be the seat of all illness.

The colon is dark, damp and warm. A perfect place for the breeding of germs and all unfriendly bacteria, as well as many parasites. It is said that it is impossible to ever gain perfect health without cleansing the colon.

– Jason Winters

Table of Contents

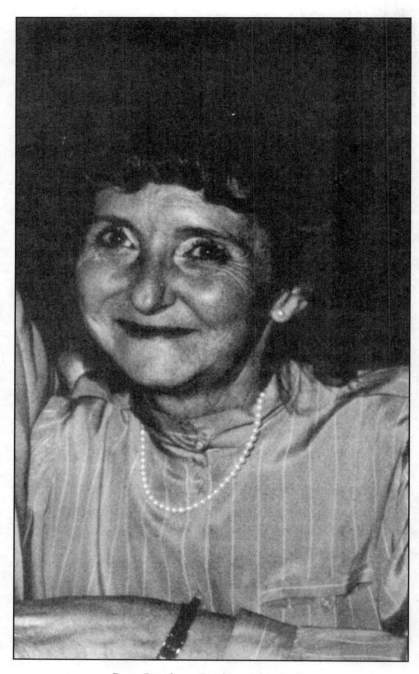

Betty Barclay – Psychic with a badge

— *1* —

BETTY BARCLAY
Faith and Love Conquers All

*I*t was a Friday night in June of 1982 when Betty was driving slowly home from a movie with her husband John. It had been a wonderful evening and they were talking softly as they proceeded through the green traffic signal. Neither of them knew that at this exact second, fate was about to deal them a terrible cruel blow, a devastating, crippling blow that would change their lives.

John was a very successful attorney in California, and Betty was a very special person also, she was psychic. Not because she wanted to be, or even studied to be, but because she was born that way. So good was she at psychic research that she was appointed the psychic consultant with the Police Department, she actually carried a badge. During the day, when not on a case, she would talk to people that called upon her for help and guidance, and the telephone counselling would take up much of her time. She was a very active woman, small and attractive, with an intense gaze that made people feel that they must be honest with her, because she would know if you were not.

A good dancer and always the center of attention she was interested in most things, her mind being always anxious to learn. Because of her visual depth perception problem, she would never drive at night, but always made John drive after sundown. This night was different, for Betty insisted that she drive. (Even she had no idea why she was so persistent.) This persistence actually saved John's life.

A car, driven by a drunk driver, roared through the red light and smashed into Betty's car with great force. Neither one of them had their seat belts fastened. Betty took the full impact of the other car, which broadsided them, hitting the door on the driver's side. It threw her against John and completely totalled the car. They both came too in the hospital, and Betty had to stay there. All of her ribs were broken, her sternum was crushed, her pelvis was fractured, she had lacerated liver, her lungs collapsed, both hips were broken and she was so bad that they kept her in the intensive care unit for twenty-five days. After the third day, her doctors told John that Betty was not going to live. Poor John had just had his spleen removed and the tail end of his pancreas that day, so one can imagine how shattering this news was to him.

Betty had stopped eating, so they had to force feed her, and drugs were impossible because her lungs were already collapsed. After twenty-five days they moved her to the surgical wing, where they said she must stay. By that time she had surprised everyone by even being alive. It was then that they told John that even if she lived, she would never walk again. The worst part, according to Betty was that she had no memory of the accident or of all the time spent in the intensive care unit. However, something kept going around in her mind, over and over again. "If they release you, and you can go home you will be alright." Day after day she pleaded with her doctor to release her, so she could go home, and one day, much against his better judgement he complied with her wishes.

She was released from the hospital in July of 1982, and as soon as she arrived home she refused to let negative thoughts enter her mind. She would pray to GOD knowing full well that HE would answer her prayer. She asked GOD to let her walk again, and she knew that HE would because she had no doubts about GOD, and her faith was extreme.

By the middle of August, that same year, six weeks later, she was slow dancing, to the utter amazement of everyone. There was no reason whatsoever that she should not be dead, but she was dancing!!

It is now 1984 and Betty is unlimited in her actions. She walks, dances, runs, and does any kind of sport she feels like. I have just heard from Betty Barclay and she is so excited, John and she are going to adopt two children and start a family.

To be able to tell you about the Betty Barclay story is a great honor for me, because it proves everything that I believe in. With everything smashed to pieces inside of her, with no health foods or medication that could help, with it being absolutely impossible for her to live, she survived to become radiantly healthy. She had the faith that GOD expected all of us to have. With that faith you need no crutches. Faith can move mountains, and that faith took Betty's frail and destroyed body and made it whole.

Her book entitled "Of Two Worlds" will be available

soon, and I hope and pray it will impart the secret of obtaining the kind of loving faith that healed Betty. A television series is also planned about her tremendous exploits aiding the police department. I called this chapter "Love Conquers All" because, the other day, Betty and John had to face this drunken driver in court. The drunken woman responsible for all the terrible agony John and Betty had gone through, did not apologize, but rather swore at them and gave them looks of hatred. When Betty was asked by the Judge a question that would either condemn or release this woman, Betty decided on the latter, and sent the woman love and understanding.

For all of you who are sick and sorrowful, please remember this story, for it is a true story, a miracle that has happened in our time.

— 2 —

INDIAN ATTACK!!

*T*he Indians had been attacking the wagon train all morning, and Audi Murphy was doing a great job picking them off, one by one. The director called for a lunch break and we all gathered around the chuck wagon – all, that is, except the Mexican Indians. They started their usual fire and began making the cactus tea they drank every day.

How we sophisticated whites would laugh at them while we gorged ourselves on jelly doughnuts, coffee with sugar and cream, and lots of cigars. I had no way of knowing that this special scene would one day, thirty years later, help to save my life. For what all these Indians were doing was purifying their blood on a daily basis, with an herbal tea.

In 1976, when I recovered from terminal cancer, I visited Tibet, the "rooftop of the world." The monastery I stayed at was populated by men all fifty years my senior, or more. I learned more from them about health, happiness and longevity than I could ever have learned from one of New York's top oncologist. For they too know about purifying the blood.

It seems that God placed a certain herb on each continent to purify a person's blood so that their natural immunity could "take care of any disease and heal the body."

God did not just throw us down here saying, "There's ten thousand fast food restaurants, go to it!" He gave us an immune system that allows the body to heal itself. However, it can't do this as long as our blood is so toxic. We have forgotten that it's natural to be healthy, and unnatural to be unhealthy. We have been brought up to believe it's the other way around. This kind of negative thinking brings about disease. Expecting to be ill causes illness.

The old man in Tibet said it quite plainly, "Tell the Americans to try expecting the best for themselves, tell them to expect a happy day, a long life and a happy one, for you create your own environment."

The art of imagery bears this out, and is now in use in alternative health clinics around the would. It has been proven that patients can "will" their immune systems to attack the illness or tumors. When it comes to cancer, however, we have a doubly hard job, for we have been so brainwashed by thinking that cancer means death. It's not their fault of course, for from birth we hear about Aunt Nellie dying of cancer, Humphrey Bogart dying of cancer, Hubert Humphrey, John Wayne, and on and on. No wonder when our white coated genius looks at us and says "cancer", we start dying right away.

The Chinese know that when all hope is taken from a person, they start dying. Tell that same person that they will live, and their body secretes certain chemicals to obey that belief. Doctors call everything that they don't understand "false hope." Well, I want to tell you that there is no such thing as false hope. Hope is faith, and faith can move mountains, so what can it do to a silly little tumor?

I know that you can probably tell me how many people die of cancer each year in America. But I bet you can't tell me how many people beat cancer and go on to live healthy, happy lives. I have made it my business to find out, and we are thousands strong.

You know, voodoo only works if the victim is told of the curse against him. His mind does the rest. He dies even though quite healthy. Following this thought, how many old movies have you seen where the doctor tells the family "We have done all we can for Aunt Nellie, the rest is up to her. She must have the will to live." Were the doctors telling us that if we had the will to live we could?

Your mind could be more powerful than you think. It could be responsible for your exact condition today, including health, wealth, and happiness. Doctors tell us that when cancer is diagnosed, they mentally write the patient off. Unfortunately so does the family and friends. Because of these negative vibrations it's pretty hard for someone still in shock over learning they have cancer to pull themselves together and prove the world is wrong, but thousands are doing it. We don't care if the medical profession calls it spontaneous remission or not. People are living and that's the bottom line.

What Has Gone Wrong?

He started by asking the above question, then without

waiting for an answer, he continued. First of all, we can't blame doctors or food manufacturers because our problems started ten thousand years ago. If our Savior had been on earth in those days, he would have been warning us of the problems involved with agriculture. At that time we changed from being hunters into herders and agriculturist. When we were hunters we had to run, stalk and skin our food and because of all this work, we did not get fat, but always stayed in top shape. If we did get fat, we could not catch our food so we did not eat, which meant we got thin so we could then run and catch our food. It is interesting to note that they had healing people even in those days. As a matter of fact, there are some historians that believe that doctors or healing persons have been around for over fifty thousand years. Because people in those days had no permanent home, they had no pollution problems. They tended to move around in groups following their food, to higher ground in the summer and so on.

It comes as a surprise to many to find out that people started using fires to cook their food well over 300,000 years ago, but as recently as 10,000 years ago cooking was only for meat and they would eat whole foods, grains, grasses, fruits and animals were consumed in their entirety. Foods consumed in their entirety seem to be balanced by nature, are healthier for the body than the food we eat today. Scientists have separated herbs, grains, etc. and the natural balance has gone. All the food in those days was alive. After all, when a tiger runs down a rabbit he does not carve off a leg and store it for next week, but rather he eats it even though the rabbit is still alive. When fish eat each other they are alive. Grains and herbs were gathered and consumed, then the people moved on to another abundant supply. They did not gather and store the food which would have meant that after a while they were eating dead food. They did not know about agriculture, the art of producing corn or wheat on the same field year after year, of using tons of fertilizers then of cutting and storing food for the future. Agriculture in this respect is bad. It showed us how to mass produce food in ground that natural chemicals and goodness has long since disappeared from. The food looks good but has very little value. Of course, nowadays, it must be sent to the supermarket to sit for weeks until we buy it. By this time it is totally dead, but something else even more deadly has been added to it along the way: preservatives. We are only now finding out how deadly this type of agriculture and preserving can be. The country that does the most of these two things, suffers the most, has far more sickness and early deaths.

Plus, don't forget the psychological effects. Ten thousand years ago it took a person only two hours each day to get enough food to fill his stomach. The rest of the time he had to himself to do whatever he wanted to. How many of us today can get by on just two hours work per day?

The food they ate was highly diversified, and it was non toxic. Anything they ate that made them feel a little sick right away, they stayed away from it in the future. The effect was immediate. Today however, due to agriculture and preservatives and dead food, the effects are slow and actually kills us over a long period of time, so that we can't place the blame on any specific thing.

For instance, if you wish to poison the mice in your house, you have to kill them the first try. If the poison just makes them sick they automatically know enough never to touch that food again.

In England they teach foxes not to attack sheep by poisoning a leg of lamb and leaving it for the fox to stumble upon. The fox gets sick and will never touch sheep again.

We in modern society have doctored up our food so that it looks good and tastes good, but in actuality, it is dead food that is slowly killing us. We have lost the natural reflex that animals still have.

With our GOD-given self healing power within each of us, it takes twenty-five years of poisoning ourselves daily for us to become ill; and because of the long time lapse, it is impossible to connect the exact cause of our degeneration and early death. One hundred years ago, 8% of our food was dead, 50 years ago 22% of the food we consumed was dead, today 75% of everything we put in our mouths is dead.

It is not only our bodies that we are destroying either, but the very air we breathe and the water we drink. If man were to cease to exist on earth today, it would take fifty years for the air alone to become pure again. It does not matter if we live in a remote farming area, for air pollution and acid rain is now everywhere.

Today we do not have the variety of foods that we had ten thousand years ago. We have the same few foods that have been made to taste different. Breakfast cereal is almost the same, yet sold under hundreds of names and flavors, all of which are dead.

In short, any food that man has fooled with is bad for you. There are well over a half a million trace additives and chemicals known to man and it is very reasonable to assume that during the course of a week we consume all of them. These trace elements are both dangerous and difficult to get rid of from your body. Has it ever occurred to you that we feed our animals better than ourselves? Look at all the signs in the zoos stating "please don't feed the animals" they are there because they don't want the animals to become ill eating such garbage.

It is wrong to say that people who enjoy health foods are going through a fad, for nothing could be further from the truth. Are they not just trying to continue the way of eating that man has become used to over fifty thousand years? By the same token, we can't say that alternative therapy is really alternative. After all, the so-called alternative therapy has been around since the beginning of man. It's medicine and drug companies which are relatively new so are in effect the alternatives.

You see, we now have to get more food per acre than we used to. Because of this we use fertilizer which contains nitrogen, potassium and phosphorous but none of the trace elements needed to make the crop nutritious. Fertilizer assists the land in producing food that looks good and in large quantities, but of extremely low nutritional value.

Our soil is deteriorating steadily, and will continue to do so. In China, however, they have managed in their own natural way of farming to keep up the quality of soil. Now, with our fertilizer and agriculture experts visiting China in order to get big sales, the soil quality of that land will quickly deteriorate. What will inevitably follow is illness of the western kind which China is at present relatively free of.

Did you know that the average American consumes over 190 lbs. of sugar each year, most of which is hidden in dead food but added just for taste, to get you and your children "hooked" on it, and all for a profit to the manufacturer. We all know that sugar is a killer. One hundred years ago the average consumption was five pounds per year. During any war there is usually a shortage of sugar, and babies born during wartime have proven far more healthy than those born at any other time.

To give you an example of the long term effect of bad food, let me state the following: Dr. Burkitt of England found that Blacks of South Africa, eating natural food had an incidence of diabetes of only three people out of forty-five thousand. The same tribe today, after consuming western food for thirty years has an incidence of diabetes amounting to fifteen thousand per forty-five thousand population.

Mr. Hoffer, that genius of nutrition, discovered that in America one third of the people admitted to a hospital were suffering from malnutrition. After seven days in the hospital however, over two thirds of the patients suffer from malnutrition. The only answer to this is to eat as little as possible while in hospital, except fruit and vegetables brought in by family and friends.

Interview with Zurich Health Magazine Aug 1984 Switzerland

I finally tracked down Jason Winters at the Palace Hotel in Bern, where I phoned for an appointment. The idea was to do a story on a man that had managed to cling to life for eight years with terminal cancer. I had read the report that he should have died seven and a half years previously.

I was not prepared for the man himself however. I met him in the lobby of the hotel, and my shock evidently showed, for Mr. Winters laughed and told me not to worry, he was used to it. I must tell the reader that I was shocked because I had readied myself to meet an old, tired sick person, underweight, with no hair, and barely clinging to life.

Jason Winters however was a giant of a man, healthy, suntanned, smiling and happy with an air of easy calmness about him. His full head of hair cut in the style that made him resemble Cary Grant. He explained to me that he jogged, lifted weights, and swam regularly.

Who would have guessed that Winters, british born, one time Hollywood stunt man, was down to only a few weeks to live back in 1977 with a massive neck tumor known as infiltrating squamous cell carcinoma? But that was three million copies of his book "KILLING CANCER" ago.

His treatment for throat, jaw and neck cancer is fully documented. His response to cobalt therapy and the suggested surgical mutilation of his neck and face are also documented.

It was because Winters suffered from the radiation therapy and was horrified at the suggested removal of his tongue, jaw bone and radical neck dissection (that may prolong his life for a few weeks) he decided to do something.

Doing something meant trips to Asia, where the Lord Buddha twenty five hundred years ago had told the Indian and Chinese people to use "herbalene" (a special herb) for their tumors. To Arizona, where the Indians have used a special herb (Chaparral) to purify their blood for centuries. And lastly to Europe where the gypsies have been using yet another herb for the same purpose, (Red Clover) - as mentioned by Jesus in the gospel of the Essenes, taken from the dead sea scrolls. Jesus evidently said, "Purify your blood with herbs and all things will fall away."

Winters, in a state of both shock and terror started reading religious books, preparing himself to meet his maker. "One thing stuck out like a sore thumb" he told me excitedly, "Herbs for health are mentioned twenty three times in our bible, and herbs for health are mentioned in absolutely every faith since the beginning of time. It was too great to be just a coincidence."

"The more I read the more the simple fact came screaming through to me. God placed an herb on each continent to do just one thing, and that is to purify a persons blood. Once a persons blood is pure, then fresh oxygen and nutrition can get to every part of the body. Suddenly a persons natural immunity starts to work and the body heals itself of disease. God did not just throw us down here and say 'There's then thousand fast food restaurants, fluoride in the water, preservatives in your food, microwave ovens, stress and war – have fun?' He gave us an immune system to fight off disease and all it needs is a little help.

When I went to Asia, North America and Europe looking for these special herbs, I found that they did not work for me until I mixed the three herbs from the three continents together. In biblical times anyone of these herbs would have worked to purify a persons blood, but that was before fluoride and junk food. Today it takes the combined efforts of the thee herbs to work."

I think that the secret message that is hidden in every religion, and has been overlooked is that "Life is in the blood. The blood of Christ" and so on. It worked for me and suddenly I started getting an awful lot of unwanted publicity about it, everyone wanted to know my story.

FORCED TO ACT

I must tell you that I was scared. I was not prepared to take on the billion dollar drug companies, The medical associations and doctors, all of whom would chew up and spit out anyone that would dare to even say that possibly, just possibly, herbs can help. Even though, of course, Hippocrates, the father of medicine told all the student doctors to use herbs for medicine.

Listen, I was just glad to be alive, I didn't want to enter a war with the biggest business in the world. They would not let me alone, however. Letters would pour in, reports on radio and T.V. kept popping up about my case. At last I gave the formula away to the Xian Corporation in England. It was kind of like giving away the formula to Coca-Cola. I had no idea that millions would soon be using it just as a kind of preventative health product.

I was amazed the other day to hear form one of England's top doctors that when I mixed the three herbs together, one of them, the herbalene, acted as a catalyst and made the other two far stronger. This was all by accident on my part because in those days I was so busy drinking and carousing and having fun that I didn't even know what a catalyst was.

THE FAMOUS AMERICAN "CHOICE" MAGAZINE,
August 1984 put it this way:

"Extensive anecdotal information has for years linked

both chaparral and red clover to anti cancer activity. Indeed, the anti cancer ingredients nordihydroguaiaretic acid-NDGA has been isolated from chaparral tea, and elixir of the American Southwest.

Herbalene may in fact be Astragalus membranaceus and Ligustrum lucidum, herbs widely used in a collective Chinese immune stimulation therapy called FU-zheng, information on which was provided, amazingly enough, in "CANCER" a publication of the American Cancer Society, in 1983; end of quote.

HERBS DO NOT CURE ILLNESS

Evidently there are millions of people in almost every country of the world taking this formula daily. It is in capsule form and is named TRIBALENE. It is already quite popular in Switzerland. I was surprised to hear Winters state the following, "I do not believe that herbs cure any illness. I believe that they merely purify the blood, and help the body get strong enough to heal itself."

Winters also surprised me further by stating that he was not against orthodox medicine and doctors; "Everyone has their place, and we must all work together for the benefit of mankind. I find doctors very helpful and understanding. Of course, we do not claim to cure anything, and if I fell down today and broke my leg I would go to the hospital immediately.

"My whole family and I have medical insurance of course, but when it comes to cancer or any other degenerative disease then I think a nutritious diet, along with special herbs help tremendously."

When I mentioned to Winters that I had read his book "KILLING CANCER" now available in the German language, and had found it fascinating reading as well as thought provoking he replied "The biggest surprise to me was when the publisher asked me to write this book, saying he would pay me twenty-six cents U.S. per copy. I thought I would be lucky to make twenty-six dollars, but as you know, its already sold nearly three million copies world wide. Even doctors are buying it for their patients that have lost all hope."

DOES NOT ALWAYS WORK

When asked if he thought that this TRIBALENE formula worked for everyone and everything, he replied "Heavens no. The biggest trouble we have is people expecting that it will and being shocked when it doesn't. For instance, someone has terminal cancer, has undergone chemotherapy and radiation, but this did no good so their doctor has sent them home to die, as a hopeless case. These people suddenly hear about Tribalene and expect it to work, in every case. Miracles do happen and a change of diet, thinking, lifestyle and blood purification often have great effects, but it is unfair to expect anything to work every time. Plus I believe that often it's just a persons time to go. On the other hand, we hear of thousands of cases of what the doctors call spontaneous remission.

HOPE AND FAITH

Winters' deep feelings of hope and faith are well worth mentioning here. I asked him if this new approach to degenerative disease would give people false hope; Winters' reply was simply "What new approach? If Jesus, Krishna, Bahaii Uhlla, Hippocrates talked about it, and if two and a half billion people of the world believe it, and have practiced it for centuries, how can you think it's new?"

He continued, "There is no such thing as false hope, for hope is faith, and faith can move mountains. If faith can move mountains then think of what it can do to a silly little tumor! Many scientists feel that when a person thinks he is going to die, their body secretes chemicals to obey that belief. On the other hand, when a person thinks he is going to live, the body secretes another type of chemical to obey that belief. You see, we are all part of God and because of that our thoughts are more powerful than you can imagine. These chemicals are called endorphins and endorcrines, and this has been proven by many people around the world. If all hope has been taken away, if you are sure you are going to die, then you will, without a doubt.

CANCER DOES NOT MEAN DEATH

People, especially in America have been brought up to believe that cancer means death. When a child, they heard that Aunt Agatha died of cancer, then John Wayne, Humphry Bogart, Hubert Humphry, Ingrid Bergman, and on and on. Naturally, when your doctor tells you that you have cancer, you start dying right away, and that's usually the end of it. I really believe in mind over matter.

Most people know that one thousand people each day die of cancer in Europe, but how many can tell us the amount of people that recovered from cancer? Not many, but I can because I have made it my business to know. There are thousands alive today that should have died, but are now back to work, leading happy healthy lives. For some strange reason they are well, in spite of everything.

I mentioned to Winters that I heard him yesterday on

a local radio show, talking through an interpreter, and had heard him say that his biggest troubles were with some born again Christians. I asked him to explain; "This is only a problem in North America. We have small groups of small minded people, living in small towns, going to a small church and listening to their small minded preacher telling them his version of the bible. His interpretation. They believe it 100%. They forget that God said "Judge not, less ye may also be judged" and also "Let he that is without sin cast the first stone." These people call anyone that does not agree with everything they say 'non-Christians.' They say that four billion people in the world are wrong, and that they are right. In fact, they cast stones at everyone. They have forgotten about watching out for false prophets, and are perfectly content to risk their eternal soul on that silly little man in the pulpit. Because their preacher does not believe in Buddha, Krishna, Bahaii Uhlla, Hippocrates, or the gospel of the Essenes, (That gospel was removed from the bible in the year 503 A.D. so that the churches would have a better hold on the congregations). All the things the world believes in, they do not. They love saying that a person is not a Christian. Their sin of judging others bothers them not at all. One day a person in their congregation with terminal cancer decided to try herbs. He had nothing to lose as he was definitely dying. He tried herbs but died anyway. Suddenly his congregation started attacking herbs and healthy diet, just because these things do not work all the time.

It is impossible to be evil without paying for it with your health, emotions and mind. Judge not means that we should not judge people. We don't need to. The spiritual people advance in perfect health and the evil ones destroy themselves.

I left Jason Winters sitting in the lobby of the hotel

sipping herbal tea with the hotel manager, and as I drove the highway back to Zurich I went over again all the things he had told me. He made no claims, he didn't believe that herbs cured disease, but rather just purified the blood, he believes in faith and eternal hope, he was a devout Christian, but most of all, he was the healthiest, tallest, most handsome person I had encountered in a long time.

The world will hear much from this man in the years ahead.

Adolph Schloss
Zuhealthmag

— 3 —

SUPPRESSED
THERAPIES

*H*ave you ever wondered what happens to all those so-called "miracle products" that receive publicity in one national newspaper or another, when you never hear of them again?

Usually the publication gets into a lot of trouble for printing it in the first place, then all future publicity is stopped. The persons selling the products are usually tricked or entrapped into a phony suit about "practicing medicine without a license" or if they can't stop them that way, they attack them on some income tax charge or other.

The following story indicates a selection of natural products that fall into the above category. Freely available in other countries, especially in socialized medicine areas, they are almost unobtainable in North America.

ERIK GUDME OF DENMARK:
A Remarkable Cancer Case

The bombs had been falling all night, and the Nazi

anti-aircraft guns had kept all of the population of Copenhagen awake.

Erik Gudme had even more problems to worry about than the bombs, for the day was April 11, 1942 and it was his day to get the results of his medical examination. He felt very ill indeed as he made his way down the Frederiksberggade to the doctor's office. His doctor was a kindly old Jewish man who had plenty of troubles of his own in this German occupied city.

The news was all bad. Erik had cancer in two places in his colon, one in the ascending colon and another growth in the descending colon. A spot on his liver looked highly suspicious, and there was a tumor the size of a small egg in his right lung. According to the doctor, the disease had been progressing for over four years. Erik's heart sank with complete and utter despair, and he cried openly in the doctor's office. The doctor went to his waiting room and sent all the other patients home, so that he could spend some time with this most distraught person.

The doctor's compassion, guidance, confidence and assurance at last penetrated Erik's fear, and thank GOD it did, for when Erik left the man's office three hours later, he took with him the information that would save his life. Erik died of natural causes in January of 1983 at the age of 85 years.

He was never to see that old Jewish doctor again, for he was killed in an explosion soon after, but he certainly lived on in Erik's mind. The information Erik received that day is still as potent and valid today, and it can really work for you, if you trust it. It is as follows:

"Don't let any man tell you when you will
is up to you, your mind and your GOD. D
man run your life. You must always remain
Never let anyone "talk" you into an operation. You must
want the operation and have faith that it will work first.
Otherwise do not have it.

Do not be overpowered by sophisticated medical men,
for more people die from the mistakes of these men than
from their illness. Remember Erik, no man can make you
do anything, for you belong only to GOD. It is quite
permissible to leave the hospital ten minutes before an
operation if you should wish to do so. Most people feel
that they are captured once in a hospital. They feel that
they must subject themselves to anything. This is wrong.
Do not hand yourself to anyone else and expect them to
cure you with a pill, for you must heal yourself. Now Erik,
eat every day four cloves of garlic, press carrots and drink
the juice. Eat or drink red clover as there is a strange
goodness in the Danish kind. (Tribalene has an abundance
of this.) Never go for a day without having a bowel
movement. Red clover or coffee enemas will clean your
colon and heal your liver. Eat no white flour, red meat or
dairy products ever again. Eat many apricot kernels each
day (15) and have lots of fruit. If you do these things Erik,
then you can live longer than I.

(The Jason Winter diet includes all of the foregoing.)

— 4 —

YUCCA

The food supplement that helps prevent and treat arthritis and high blood pressure.
by Shideler Harpe

"We've known for several years that a food supplement extracted from yucca can be remarkably effective in preventing, eliminating and reducing the pain, swelling and joint stiffness suffered by arthritis victims. Now there is indisputable evidence that this natural plant substance can prevent and lower high blood pressure, high cholesterol, and high triglyceride levels in the blood. We seem to only have scratched the surface of the medical uses of yucca."

–Robert Bingham, M.D.
"Arthritis News Today"

THE NATION'S estimated 50 million arthritis victims received encouraging news four years ago when a medical team reported that a natural plant substance had proven effective in relieving the pain, stiffness and swelling of some kinds of arthritis. Doctors reported that a food supplement, an extract made from the yucca plant, contained a natural substance which often acted like cortisone on the swelling and pain of arthritis, but it did not cause any unpleasant or harmful side effects.

In a twelve-month controlled study at the National Arthritis Medical Clinic in Desert Hot Springs, California, doctors found more than 60% of the 149 patients monitored by the medical team reported varying degrees of relief of pain, stiffness and swelling of arthritis without any ill effects whatsoever. Further testing in 1978-79 has confirmed findings of the previous report and also has indicated that the yucca treatment can benefit patients suffering from hypertension and from symptoms of abnormally high cholesterol and triglycerides in the blood.

Favorable results were achieved after administration of the food supplement containing the yucca steroid saponin in tablet form, according to Dr. Robert Bingham, an orthopedic surgeon, founder and director of the National Arthritis Medical Clinic, who also has an arthritis and orthopedic practice in Yorba Linda, California.

Since Dr. Bingham's first report in 1975 called attention to the efficacy of yucca in treating arthritis, other physicians in Southwestern states and elsewhere have included yucca extract tablets in their regimen of treatment for arthritic disease. Their independent findings confirm Dr. Bingham's original conclusion that yucca extract is beneficial in treating these widespread diseases. Dr. Bingham's newest report on the effects of yucca upon high blood pressure and other health problems has been greeted with great interest and continues to be the subject of further clinical trials.

Results of the Study

In the patient population, 64.6% were female and 34.5% were male. Osteoarthritis accounted for 58.9% of cases and rheumatoid arthritis for 41.1%. The disease had been present from 2 months to 42 years, with an average of 14.6 years.

The food supplement tablets were taken before, during, and after meals – 2 tablets, 3 times a day – with no problems reported. The yucca concentrate proved to be non-irritating to the gastrointestinal tract. Some patients reported less gas and constipation.

Improvement in arthritis. 49% felt less pain, stiffness, and swelling, the three major complaints of arthritis. This suggests that the normal intestinal flora of beneficial microscopic plant life may indeed be under stress in arthritis patients. The study concludes that yucca extract benefits normal bacterial forms in the alimentary canal.

Researchers considered it important that "no allergic manifestations appeared." This was not surprising, since yucca has served as a food for thousands of years. This seems to confirm evidence that the active principal, yucca saponin, is not absorbed into the blood but works within the small and large intestines. Its benefits are in the improvement and protection of intestinal flora rather than any direct action upon the arthritis.

There is strong evidence that some forms of arthritis may be caused or worsened by toxic substances in the intestines and that these toxins may be absorbed by the body. Most patients who report a reduction of swelling and stiffness in their joints are patients who suffer gastrointestinal disturbances associated with arthritis.

Yucca pills seem to inhibit pathological bacteria and protozoa that occur in the intestines. They also seem to help the natural and normal forms of bacteria found in the tract. Since there is very little or no absorption into the body, a patient does not need to worry about drug reactions or a conflict between yucca and other medication.

Since the publication of his original report, Dr. Bingham has continued to use yucca as a food supplement in the treatment of about 2,000 arthritis patients. Other physicians have added the yucca extract to their treatment regimens. Impressive results have been reported by Dr. Paul Isaacson of Tucson, Arizona and Dr. Robert A. Elliott of Woodland Hills, California.

Dr. Isaacson reports that "the treatments are relieving the patient's discomfort and sometimes the swelling. I would say that 90% of my patients have gotten relief to some degree ... before using yucca I just didn't get the results I'm getting now."

Dr. Elliott says that "about 50% of my patients have gained some relief from arthritis symptoms while taking the yucca tablets," and he noted that "yucca therapy seems to have a role in reducing cholesterol and triglyceride levels in the blood."

Details of the 1978 Study

Dr. Bingham's 1975 report first noted that use of yucca in treating arthritis resulted in several unexpected side effects — lowering of blood pressure, relief from headaches, reduction of blood cholesterol levels, and reduction of blood triglyceride levels. Additional studies appeared to be in order. Accordingly, 212 patients with high blood pressure and high cholesterol levels were given either yucca extract tablets or a placebo tablet in a random selection double-blind study: 124 patients suffered from osteoarthritis, and 88 had rheumatoid arthritis.

Each patient received a complete orthopedic examination, blood count, blood chemistry, and sedimentation rate tests. All patients were placed on high-protein diets stressing natural foods and vitamin supplements. They participated in exercise and physical therapy programs. During the study, all of the patients showed some improvement.

A random selection was used, neither the doctor nor patient knowing which tablet was given. Office nurses were the only ones who knew which patients received the placebo. The information was kept confidential until completion of the study. All patients were informed that the first tablets they would receive **might** be placebos or **might** be yucca tablets. They also were told that, if they were given the placebo, their treatment would be changed to the yucca tablets.

Results of the Test

As in the original study, the medical team again found that about two-thirds of the patients received some benefit from taking yucca extract. Non had any unpleasant reactions, complication, or ill effects from using yucca.

The 212 patients participating in the study were divided into three groups. The first group of 36 patients received the placebo tablets only. These were identical in appearance, color, size, and taste to the yucca tablets, but contained **none** of the yucca extract. A second group of 138 patients received **only** the yucca tablets. A third group of 38 patients was given the placebo for 1 or 2 months, then received yucca tablets for 1 to 6 months, or more. The average patient took the yucca tablets, or a liquid extract of equivalent potency, for 6 months to a year.

Results. Blood pressures were reduced, on the average, 13 mm/Hq in the placebo groups (who were on diet and exercise therapy); 24mm/Hq in the yucca treated group. Blood cholesterol was reduced 40mg/100ml in the placebo groups; 110mg/100ml in the yucca group. Triglycerides were reduced 17mg/100ml in the placebo groups; 24mg/100ml in the yucca group.

Dr. Bingham's report on these three factors show the results from the yucca treatment were greater than the reductions with placebos, diet, and exercises.

Dr. Bingham also suggests that yucca saponin may tend to break down the high molecular fats in foods whose absorption contributes to high blood pressure, hardening of the arteries, hypertriglyceridemia, and hypercholesterolemia.

One of the doctor's most significant findings was that **no patient on yucca extract for 6 months or more continued to show an abnormally high blood pressure or excessive blood triglyceride and cholesterol levels.** In other words, there were permanent benefits from the period of yucca therapy.

Certainly, the wild desert cactus plant known as the yucca is a natural benefactor to mankind.

PREVENTION AND TREATMENT OF ARTHRITIS

"Yucca plant saponin in the management of Arthritis." This food supplement, extracted from the desert Yucca plant, has now been used in over 2,000 cases. It is a plant steriod substance, not absorbed in the intestines, which has a beneficial effect, helping to eliminate pathogenic organisms and plant forms, and reduce intestinal symptoms and disorders which are present in so many patients with arthritis. Besides less stiffness and soreness in the joints, which was the most frequent benefit of the treatment, many patients experience a relief of constipation, intermittent diarrhea, cramping, abdominal pains, intestinal gas, a lessening of headaches of the migraine type, and the blood picture of these patients showed a lowering of abnormal cholesterol levels.

IN SUMMARY: Newer treatment methods include the use of Yucca as a food supplement, arthritis vaccines to improve the patient's immunity to infections, and anti-protozoal drugs should be given to patients with acute and active rheumatoid arthritis. Surgical replacement of joints destroyed by arthritis is safer and more successful after the patient has been on this type of medical and nutritional management for a month or more. The approach of Dr. Wyburn-Mason to the treatment of rheumatoid arthritis, for the first time in medical history, makes improvement and the arrest of this disease a predictable result. The use of megavitamin therapy and minerals, particularly vitamin A, D, calcium, are essential to rebuilding of the bone and joint structures in arthritis patients. Further progress in the treatment of all forms of arthritis and prevention of most arthritic diseases are based on applied nutrition, exercise and careful medical management.

BIBLIOGRAPHY

1. *Bingham, Robert – "Nutrition in the Treatment of Arthritis," Journal of Applied Nutrition, Vol. 25, pg. 112-125, Winter 1972*

2. *Bingham, Robert; Bellew, Bernard A.; and Bellew, Joeva G., "Yucca Plant Saponin in the Management of Arthritis." Journal of Applied Nutrition, Vol. 27, No. 2 & 3, pg. 45-50. Fall, 1975.*

3. *Bingham, Robert – "Rheumatoid Disease. Has One Investigator Found its Cause and Cure?" The work of Dr. Roger Wyburn-Mason, Modern Medicine, pg. 38-47, February 15, 1976.*

— 5 —

FLUORIDE AND THE GOVERNMENT LAW SUIT

*I*n the latter part of 1983 an elderly lady living in Scotland found fluoride in her city drinking water. She was so upset that she took the Scottish government to court for putting poison in the water, and she won.

It is well to note that fluoride is against the law in many countries because it is a health hazard. It has also never been proven that fluoride reduces cavities. As one doctor said, after visiting the United States: "Even if fluoride did reduce cavities, who would want to full set of teeth long after you have died of cancer."

Fluoride is such a big business in America, they have even got the dentists washing our mouths out with it. It's called double exposure now. You know, the dentist keeps telling you that his x-ray machine is too weak to give you cancer, so now they have added fluoride to their treatment, something just as dangerous.

With constant advertising for fluoride tooth paste, and fluoride also in all of our drinking water it's no wonder that people from other countries shudder at the dangerous life we are living.

One Englishman told me that he can remember when it was the Mexican water that was not safe to drink, now the joke is to tell people planning to visit America, "It's a great place but don't drink the water."

Fortunately many groups of knowledgeable people have started demonstrating about this great threat to human life, and they also need your support. Don't let anyone say it's just in minute quantities, because you are already getting minute quantities of about 2,000 things each day that are dangerous, and they do add up.

I understand that there are two brands of toothpaste on the market without fluoride. They are McLean's and Pepsodent. If you want to survive the drinking water problem, you need a reverse osmosis machine, not a filter or bottled water, which are sometimes worse.

PUREST WATER AVAILABLE

Pure water is the greatest necessity for all forms of life, and yet today it is almost impossible to obtain. The additives used by the water departments are doing us almost as much damage as would the untouched polluted water.

Water distillers are great, but expensive. Reverse osmosis, I feel is the answer, as it takes no machine to operate, and no electrical power. The reverse osmosis water purifier costs less than half of the regular water distiller. Reverse osmosis developed by the U.S. Department of Interior License #3417870 is the finest home water purification process available. Purwater systems typically removes 95% of total dissolved solids plus all bacteria, pesticides, asbestos, radiation, organics, dissolved gasses, virus, turbidity, discoloration, amoebae, custs, spores, and reduces suspected cancer-causing organic chemicals, like trihalomethanes (THMs), Carbon tetrachloride, benzene, PCB's to safe levels.

How does this marvelous system work? Polluted water is forced by water pressure against a semi-permeable membrane. Purified water molecules easily pass through the membrane, while pollutants cannot pass though and are washed down the drain.

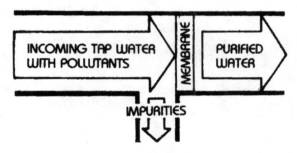

Improve the quality of your life through the quality of your water. Address for information appears in back of book.

— 6 —

COBALT RADIATION POISONING

*I*f you have been subjected to cobalt radiation and/or x-rays then you are suffering a little from radiation poisoning. It's no accident that doctors and nurses disappear behind lead doors while they bombard you with rays.

Here's how to get rid of the ill-effects.

Pour one pound of pure salt purchased from a health store (not iodized), and one pound of baking soda, into a hot bath and stay in the water for twenty minutes. Immerse the part affected if possible. Do this twice each week for one month. If you have any surgical scars or radiation burns, spread on vitamin E liberally over the affected parts.

EXERCISING AND LOSING WEIGHT

*T*here are many benefits from a good exercise program, and some of them are a reduction of fatigue, more energy, better thinking, improved circulation and lowering of high blood pressure in many instances. It dispels despair and anxiety, and we feel sure, helps the body fight off such things as heart troubles and cancer. The exercise program must be used in conjunction with a good diet of at least 50% live food, such as fruit, vegetables and nuts.

You do not need to enter into a heavy exercise program, but rather something that you can stay with for life, something that you feel comfortable with. I lift free weights each day, cycle three miles, do sit ups and end up each morning with a sauna and ice cold plunge in the special plunge tank. Then I feel ready to tackle the world. I do this after drinking one pint of lemon juice at room temperature.

Regular exercise changes the metabolism of your body, lowering body fats such as lipoprotein cholesterol, which if allowed to build up pre-disposes you to all kinds of

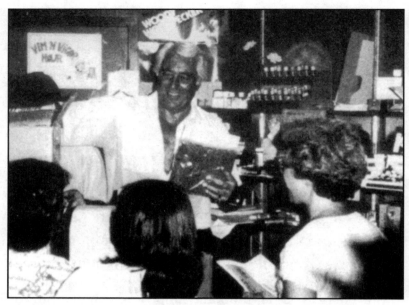

Live Radio in Hawaii

artery and heart troubles. It also possibly helps prevent the accumulation of fats in the arteries.

I believe that you must combine exercise and diet. If you must diet alone then your metabolism slows down also, so you burn less calories and so have a harder time losing weight than if you were eating normally but exercising considerably.

Vigorous exercise will offset the slow down of your metabolism and will hasten the weight loss without making you feel depressed. Did you know that mild exercise actually reduces your appetite?

Because muscle weighs more than fat, it is quite possible that you may not lose pounds, but will lose many inches. Do not worry about the weight as you are just "redistributing" your body, and turning fat into muscle. People will remark that you must have lost thirty pounds when actually it was only ten pounds but that was fluid that makes you look old and bloated in all the wrong places.

Isometric Exercises: Pushing and straining your muscles against immovable objects. The best exercises in the world are isometric. You can do them anywhere, and you don't need to buy expensive equipment. Set aside twenty minutes each day, except Sunday, and do sit ups, push ups, leg lifts – then lean against the wall and push with your back, as though you are pushing a car. Now push the wall with your hands (facing the wall). You must exert yourself, and don't overdo it, just try to do a little bit better each week. The results will astound you. Try to walk at least one and a half miles a day.

Health spas and gymnasiums make their money out of the "spur of the moment" people who suddenly have the urge to better themselves, so they buy a lifetime membership in a club, go just two or three times, then never return. If every member showed up at the same time, the place would not be able to hold a tenth of them, inmost cases.

Also, many homes have closets full of exercise equipment, purchased once again on the spur of the moment, and rarely if ever used. That is why it is better to return once again to the simple way of exercising, as outlined above. After all, you already own a wall, so why bother with anything else.

Before you start any exercise program, stretch your body, like a cat does upon waking. You have to get flexibility into your muscles before you start. A cat never wakes up and starts dashing around as we do when our alarm sounds in the morning. He lays and stretches his legs, back, and neck, and this is what we should also do prior to getting out of bed. You can set your alarm for five minutes earlier, and that will give you enough time to make yourself supple and flexible.

— 8 —

ALCOHOLISM

When a person is healing people and is not a medical doctor, does not belong to the A.M.A., and if he is not prescribing harmful drugs, then he can expect to be persecuted.

So it was with some concern that the staff of one clinic was shaken when the stranger standing bleary-eyed in the middle of the waiting room said, "I have a very responsible position and need help."

Dr. Oswald saw him at once and soon found out that the man was an alcoholic to the extent he was about to lose everything, career, home and family.

Quite used to helping friends and enemies alike, Dr. Oswald told him, "The only way for an alcoholic to be cured is for him to want to be cured." The man said that he wanted to be free of this thing that was destroying his life, more than anything else in the world, so Oswald started him on the following program.

First came the colon cleanse mentioned earlier, and so important as the first step in any recovery. Next came the phosphates that fed the man's nervous system constantly. Then the correcting of the chronic imbalances created by the alcohol. Once this step is completed then all craving for alcohol disappears. The patient is then taken off of all sugar and sugar-based foods. And special liver rebuilding tablets are administered.

In this man's case the treatment only took two weeks to become totally effective, but Dr. Oswald emphasizes the point that during that time the person must be worked with very closely. It is not as effective if a person is just sent home with the information in order to do it all himself. He needs the encouragement and help of a trained person on a twenty-four hour basis. When I took up this point with Hanne Kramb, she said her therapy was the same except that she had found certain pressure points on the ear that allows the patient to take quicker advantage of the therapy.

Mr. Rolf Effern, Hanne's pharmacist and licensed chemist told us of a certain herb now available that prohibits an alcoholic from drinking, for each time he does he becomes very sick to the stomach. The difficulty, of course, is getting the patient to take the herbal formula each day.

SERGEANT BORKOWSKI ATHLETE'S FOOT

*I*n Poland the enlisted men suffered terribly from athlete's foot, which is highly contagious. This uncomfortable scourge spread through the camps like the plague.

Sergeant Borkowski came from the town of Lodz, a hundred miles from Warsaw, and upon reviewing his service record with a view to promotion, the group of examining officers found that the Sergeant had never suffered from any foot ailment during his seventeen years of service, not even the very common athlete's foot.

This discovery caused great excitement for if the man had a secret remedy or preventative for this, it would be worth a fortune, plus would be of great benefit to the whole army.

It was with great embarrassment that Borkowski stood in the health officer's board room, and in front of seven other officers was forced to explain exactly what he did to avoid foot problems.

It was simply that each morning, while taking a shower, Borkowski urinated on his feet, just as his old father had told him to do. There was certainly no glamour here, and no money to be made, but the information was officially passed around to others. It seems, upon careful study, that urine has thousands of antibodies that are most effective in fighting infections.

It was with enormous embarrassment to the Canadian Television Network when they interviewed a high Indian official from New Delhi on live television, seen by hundreds of thousands of viewers, the announcer, a very proper individual asked the Indian to what he credited his good health and excellent skin, to which he quickly replied, "I drink my own urine." I suppose that it would be hard to gain your composure after an answer like that. He was not joking, of course. Many investigations have been done pertaining to mare's urine as it seems to give the immune system a giant boost, but somehow I don't think the western world will ever accept that. I can imagine the look on a bleary-eyed patient's face when he looks up at you from his bed and says, "What is this stuff I am drinking, anyway?" and you tell him!!

— 10 —

COLDS, CATTARH AND THE ROMAN ARMY

*B*efore going on long marches, or into battle, the Roman army were fed a small amount of garlic each day. This would ward off colds, plus give the soldiers strength and stamina. The gladiators were fed massive steaks, done very rare, along with garlic cloves. The meat was to bring out their anger and ferocity in the arena and the garlic would give them strength and cause the fight to last much longer.

Down through the centuries garlic has been well known as a quick remedy for colds and cattarh. In many countries it is used as a necklace worn by people with sore throats or bad head or chest conditions. The strange thing is that if someone wears a garlic necklace, and they have a sore throat, the strength of the garlic quickly diminishes. But if you wear one and are healthy, then the garlic retains its strength for many days. chewing a small piece of garlic purifies the teeth, gums, tongue and throat, rids the intestines of parasites and mucus, right down to the colon.

It is peculiar that we pull away from someone who has

just eaten garlic, which should be a sign to us that they have just purified their body, yet we gladly hug and kiss someone that has just finished a hamburger and milk shake, loading their intestines with thick green putrid mucus. If you live in a cold damp climate, then to avoid colds, bronchitis, asthma and sore throats just crush up two vitamin C tablets (1000 mg), mix it with hot water and let it trickle down your throat. Follow with a garlic piece and you can breathe better right away. Very unscientific, but as long as it works, what does it matter.

— 11 —

DYSENTERY AND THE BRITISH OFFICER

When the British army were fighting the Dervishes and the Fuzzy Wuzzies in Africa, the most common complaint among the soldiers and officers alike was stomach problems, due to the drastic change of water, diet and weather. The same thing happened to the soldiers serving in the Khyber Pass area of India. After exhausting large supplies of medicine that did not work, a captain in the medical corps found that if you placed one ounce of port wine and one ounce of brandy into a glass and sipped on it, then repeated the procedure every three hours, the problem would disappear in every case.

The trouble with this, however, was that when the regular soldiers learned about this treatment, there soon appeared a line up outside the dispensary, with all the men claiming upset stomachs.

I have learned from visiting friends in Acapulco that it is also very effective against Montezuma's revenge.

— 12 —

GALLSTONES

*H*ere is what a top American nutritionist told me to do about this, simply and easily without surgery.

My whole family has done this successfully.

Drink one quart of apple juice daily for five days. This will soften up the stones to such an extent that you could squash them in your fingers.

On the sixth day, skip dinner and at 6p.m. take a tablespoonful of epsom salts with water. Repeat at 8 p.m. At 10 p.m. make a cocktail of four ounces of olive oil and four ounces of fresh squeezed lemon juice. Shake vigorously and drink right down. In the morning you will pass green stones varying from the size of grains of sand to some as large as your thumb nail. You won't feel a thing, but will be amazed at the results. Thousands have done this instead of major surgery.

— 13 —

TEA TREE OIL

*"H*is hands became like velvet in one week" said the physician. He was referring to a bad case of fungus infection on the hands of a young boy on which the usual medications had failed, but which had responded remarkably to this new wonder oil in one (1) week. AUSTRALIAN TEA TREE OIL. This occurred in a modern clinic in the Great Boston Area, Massachusetts. This physician is now trying it in the treatment of other conditions. Scores of equally amazing reports come from Australian practitioners who have used the powerful healing oil now for many years. From whence does it come?

Tea Tree Oil comes from the interior of Australia, principally from the North Rivers country of New South Wales. As its name indicates, it is produced from the Tea Tree, but there are hundreds of kinds of tea trees in Australia. This antiseptic oil comes from only one species known as Molaleuea Alternifolis. It grows in swampy areas and is so hardy that it cannot be readily wiped out and the swamps drained or redeemed. To destroy it the very roots must be pulled out of the soil. The oil is distilled by steam from the leaves and branch-lets, a thousand pounds of these yielding only eighteen (18) pounds of oil. This oil is a light straw color or it may be water white. Both of these types are frequently used in therapeutic work. Out of some 300 species only one shows the now famous antiseptic and healing properties. In Australia it is widely used by doctors and dentists as well as in many products sold to the public for home antisepsis and healing.

Tea Tree Oil has gained its reputation from the fact that it is more powerful in its action than carbolic acid and at the same time in non-irritating to sensitive tissues, and absolutely non-poisonous. (This makes it a wonderful antiseptic to use where there are children). It is remarkably healing and many doctors report that it heals frequently without even permitting a scar to remain. It is applied in its pure state, or diluted to various percentages with bland oils; as an ointment; and as emulsified or saponified solution which is miscible with water in all proportions; the more usual percentages marketed, however, being: 40%, 20%, or 5% strength.

Among the many conditions treated we find perinychia, empyema, gynaecological conditions, skin conditions (such as impetigo contagiousm), pediculosis, ringworm, tinea, athlete's foot, acute nasopharyngitis, catarrh, thrush, "aphethous" stomatitis, tonsillitis, sore throat, and ulcers of the mouth. It is most helpful in treating scratches, insect bites, itches, sores, wounds and abrasions of the everyday type, pimples, boils and carbuncles. In fact, it is excellent for boils or carbuncles since it is easily applied straight, penetrating right into the boil or carbuncle, mixing with the puss and causing cleansing and healing to take place. Its remarkable healing action is due to the characteristic it has of mixing with pus and necrosed tissue in wounds giving germicidal action and sloughing away of the dead and evil tissue while leaving a healthy, unirritated, healing surface. Because of these properties, during World War II it was widely used in British machine shops mixed with cutting oils to reduce the absenteeism caused by infections occurred by cuts and scratches from metal edges and so forth. In the South Pacific men rubbed themselves with it to keep away the mosquitoes and other insects.

It is now widely used by Australian dentists for work on pyorrhea, to swab out cavities and to clean up pus pockets in general. It's action is swift, effective and at the same time it serves as a deodorant, itself having a very pleasant sort of spicy and nutmeg smell.

When tested on typhoid bacillus it killed off in thirty seconds. This was only a 2 ½ % solution. The 100% pure oil is used for painting carbuncles, boils and pimples; for ringworm–tropical ringworm and tinea; internally for colitis, root canal treatment and as an inhalant for coryza. It can be blended with bland oils to produce many desired strength. Such oils as olive, corn, cottonseed or peanut may be used. Five percent (5%) mixed with light paraffin oil (mineral oil) makes a fine nose and throat spray. It is used full strength for pyorrhea, swabbing out tooth sockets after extractions, injecting into unbroken boils and for insect bites. It is wonderful for dirty and foul wounds. It deodorizes, cleans and heals. This same strength is used for mouth ulcers, necorsed alveolus sloughing and open or exposed ulcers (external). A solution of this in water is used for abscessed cavities, gingivitis, mouth wash, halitosis-suppurations, impetigo or septic throat. For gonorrhea and for vaginal douches a 1% solution of this 40% strength emulsified solution in water is recommended.

Now we will quote directly from reports by Australian practitioners just to give a more detailed picture of how they apply this:

• "Colitis with hemorrhage cured in two weeks. Bowel washed out with a 1% solution frequently and 5 drops of the pure oil 3 times a day taken internally."

• "Suppurating bruise of shin which appeared to be progressing to a condition of periostitis, checked in 24 hours using solution diluted 1 to 40 as a compress. Condition cured in one week by continuing this treatment."

• "The condition called 'Erosion of the Cervix' has been one of the bug-bears of general practice. Much surgery has been performed and much ink has been spilled, but the general practitioner still has the female patient with an "issue" of mucopurulent material of many years standing. In these two cases tried, the issue has stopped and remained stopped for two months. If this Tea Tree Oil solution will perform this miracle it will soon have more than an Australian reputation ..."

• "Pruritic acne, which patient said was very worrying, cleared with one wash of this solution after he had had a bath."

• "For superficial cuts, bruises and small contusions the oil is painted on 100% and left to dry, a scab forms and healing under the scab almost invariably takes place within a few days."

• "Superficial burns and scalds are very common with sugar boilers and as a first dressing the 40% solution is painless and soothing, and later on, the deeper burn, if suppuration occurs, a dressing 1 to 40 or 1 to 20 is clean and satisfactory."

For **stiffened, sore joints** or tendonitis, apply the Tea Tree Oil before taking a steam bath or while taking a sauna, directly on the affected joints. It is extremely effective to apply the oil while lying in the sun which helps draw it into the tissues. A doctor in Hawaii tells us he has success using Tea Tree Oil on his patients with **blurred vision,** applying it to the forehead and cheek area while lying in the sun. A doctor in Texas treats many different disorders – **tennis elbow, achilis tendon, bursitis** – by applying Tea Tree Oil while patients are under a sun or heat lamp.

• "Personally free from colds during the year – previously unknown. Personal friends relieved and cured or head and chest flu by inhaling (1) from a teaspoon of the pure oil in a pint of boiling water, or (2) inserting a little of the pure oil in the nostril frequently."

It is useful internally as a stimulating expectorant in chronic laryngitis and bronchitis, and is stated to be useful as an anthelmintic, especially against the roundworm. It's most frequent uses, however, are externally in the treatment of various skin diseases. For this latter group of affections it is used for its antiparasitic effect in such diseases as scabies, trinea versicolor, etc., and for its stimulation action in acne rosaceae, psoriasis, and other chronic conditions. It is also used externally as a counter-irritant in chronic rheumatism and other painful conditions.

— 14 —

THE KIDNEYS

W hen it comes to taking good care of the kidneys, I found it very strange that people from over thirty countries that I visited all had the same old ancient remedy. They claim this simple remedy was passed down to them by their forefathers who always knew just what to do with any kidney problem.

As we have discussed, your body can heal itself, providing you give it a chance, so the first thing you have to do to help the kidneys is simply to "flush them out." Once this is done to mother nature's satisfaction, then the healing is very quick.

Each morning, squeeze one whole lemon into a pint of warm water, (distilled if possible) and drink it down. It goes straight to the kidneys and starts its purifying and healing. No sugar allowed!

Apart from this, what a wonderful way to start the day, with a good old fashioned vitamin health drink, instead of that terrible coffee that aids in screwing up the kidneys.

— 15 —

EMPHYSEMA

*T*here is a combination of herbs developed by the Health Centers that has proven so effective in cases such as asthma and emphysema, that it defies description. It is known as "detox" soon to be available world wide.

I had been smoking twenty ciggs each day ever since I was fourteen years of age. In 1976 I had asthma so bad that I could not run anymore, or even walk fast. In bed I had to be propped up with pillows so that I could sleep. Up until this time I had always been very active. I made the same old silly excuses that all smokers make. It was just a cold, I was allergic to something, I will be better next week, it's good to have all the mucus in your lungs as it's bad if they are bone dry. The day came however, when I had an appointment with Dr. Agnew of Prince George, Canada. He listened carefully to my breathing through his stethoscope then said, "Haw, Haw, Haw. Do you ever have emphysema!!!" Suddenly all of my stupid excuses went right down the drain. I had emphysema bad. "Do you mind if I have a cigarette right now, doctor?" Whenever I was scared I smoked. "Not at all," he said and he made out a prescription. "Of course it will do nothing but get worse from now on. There is really nothing anyone can do because your lungs have lost the elasticity necessary for you to breathe."

Six months later, still smoking heavily, I was told that I had terminal cancer, with only three months to live. This certainly was not one of my better years. As I have said, that was seven years ago and just to prove a point, I entered a weight-lifting contest last year for people over forty years of age and I won. I can and do often run five miles and I work out at the health spa each day.

I did it all by following GOD'S rules and regulations. Diet, herbs, (Tribalene) and proper thinking. No one can ever tell me that an illness is terminal, and they can never take away all my hope and faith, for by letting them do this, they might just as well shoot you on the spot. The results are just the same.

When you are sent home to die by your doctor, the only thing to do is either die or try what they call alternative therapies. It is the establishment that dares to call nutrition, herbalism, etc. "alternative therapies". I prefer to call the comparatively new orthodox medicine the alternative therapy, for after all, diet, nutrition and herbs have been curing people for thousands of years. The so-called orthodox therapy is relatively something new.

It doesn't mention anything about cutting, chemotherapy and radiation in the Bible. Buddha never spoke of it, neither did Jesus. Maybe they thought it wasn't worth speaking about.

The question is, "what on earth are we going to do with all these terminal patients that refuse to terminate?"

They are out there by the thousands and their numbers are growing. It is a terrible embarrassment for a doctor to send someone home to die with no hope whatsoever, only to find him living healthily years later.

Imagine how the New York doctor felt after sending Paul Vendon home to die with only two months to live. Then years later while on a vacation in Florida, the doctor jumps into a cab only to find it being driven by the terminal patient – suntanned, robustly healthy. While the doctor had that unhappy pallor common to his profession.

The driver explained that after leaving the doctor's office with the death sentence, he moved down to Florida to spend his last days. He lay out in the sun, met a group of vegetarians and in spite of his great faith in the doctor, he just started feeling too good to die. He has since married a beautiful Miami blonde and they have a very fine son.

You cannot treat just one part of your body. It has to be the whole thing or nothing. This is the wholistic approach and I can't for the life of me understand why people fight this simple approach to good health. It's in every scripture and in any library. Some experts say that the real true way to excellent health is so easy, that people can't accept it. If it doesn't involve drugs and mutilation, loss of savings and terribly difficult terms, then it just could not work.

The truth is always simple. The North American Indians did not spend billions of dollars each year on research to know that chaparral is a great blood purifier. It certainly is and they use it daily.

The Russian lumber jacks did not spend millions on

74

nd pay scientists high salaries to tell them that obed D.M.S.O. on their swollen hands the pain arthritis would go. They still use it every day.

The gypsies of Europe did not spend billions to find out that Red Clover is a great medicine and blood purifier. By consuming it they recover from illnesses, including asthma and lung problems, and feel great.

We always take the most difficult way, and if something is any good, then it's got to be very expensive and can be obtained only by prescription.

ELECAMPANE
(Inula Helenium COMPOSITAE)

Elecampane's properties are beneficial to all pulmonary and catarrhal affections. Its sodium phosphate cleans the liver and digestive organs, the potassium chloride dissolves the fibrinous exudations and mucoid matter, and its calcium chlorine supports, feeds, and tones the heart muscles. It is a stimulant, a relaxant, and a tonic to the mucous membrane (a warming, strengthening, cleansing and toning agent to the gastic, alvine and pulmonary membranes). Because of its powerful healing action and efficient expectoration of pulmonary mucus, some herbalists have considered this agent specifically for consumption and pulmonary disorders. It promptly clears up old chronic diseases of the lungs and chest. This herb is the richest source of insulin (a carbohydrate).

Medicinal uses: Cough, asthma, bronchitis, all pulmonary complaints, dyspepsia, acute catarrhal affection, tuberculosis, snake bites, cyspnea or shortness of breath, wheezing, cystitis, skin diseases, inflammations (all forms), putrid sores and cankers, rash (skin and face), tooth decay, whooping cough, dropsy, diptheria, kidney and bladder stones, retention of urine, delayed menstruation, (amenorrhea), phthisis, vesical catarrh, sluggish liver, kidney problems, bowel problems, ulcers, malnutrition, rickets, glandular insufficiency, nervous debility, and muscular weakness.

Skin

Putrid sores, cancers, and rash: Apply the agent externally as a fomentation poultice, ointment, or wash.

HOREHOUND
(Marubium vulgare; LABITATAE)

Common names: Horehound, hoarhound, white horehound, common horehound, marubium and marrubio (Span.).

Identifying characteristics:
Stem: Square, covered with white and wooly hair (tomentose), spreading branches, numerous stems, 1-2 feet high, bushy and leafy.

Leaves: Cordate (heart-shaped) and roundish-ovate, opposite 3/5 - 2 inches long, coarsely crenate, crinkly, gray-green, blunt-toothed, rough (strongly rugose-veined), power petioled, upper sessile, and white-hairy.

Flowers: Small and whitish or cream colored, tubular, in dense auxiliary whorls just above the upper leaves, 10-toothed, calyxerect- spreading and pungent.

Root: Fibrous, shot rootstock and exudes a persistent bitter acid.

Taste: Aromatic and bitter, but pleasant.

Odor: Characteristic (distinct).

Part used: Herb.

Therapeutic action: Expectorant, tonic, stomachic, diaphoretic, bitter, slightly diuretic, emmenagogue, pectoral, aromatic, hepatic, resolvent, stimulant, cathartic (large doses), anthelmintic (vermifuge), and culinary.

Horehound is probably the most popular of <u>the herbal remedies to the respiratory system.</u> It is taken most frequently in the lozenge or cough drop form. It is quite effective for all pulmonary complaints as an expectorant, tonic and diaphoretic. As a mild diaphoretic, horehound will promote profuse perspiration and will relieve the hyperemic conditions of the lungs and other congestions by promoting a gentle outward flow of the blood. It has been highly valued as a soothing expectorant for at least 350 years. Culpepper wrote that "it helpeth to expectorate tough phlegm from the chest". As an emmenagogue agent, in case of abnormal absence or suppression of the menstrual discharge (amenorrhea), it will regulate the flow and in parturition, it will assist the expulsion of afterbirth.

Medicinal uses: Hoarseness, coughs, asthma, cough, pulmonary troubles, amenorrhea, croup, chest colds, congestion, dyspepsia, jaundice, hysteria, expelling of worms, chronic sore throat, tuberculosis, dyspnea or difficult breathing, constipation, suppressed urine, chronic rheumatism, colic, stomach ache, intermittent fever, pneumonia, chronic hepatitus, phthisis, cachexia, and catarrh.

— *16* —

TENSION CAN MAKE YOU ILL
– Cancer help Center

*I*n the history of mankind, there may never have been a time when individuals were free from the challenging circumstances that life presents in some form or other. Today, we are certainly conscious of tremendous pressures which seem to assail us from all directions and which so often contribute to tension both in body and mind.

During stressful conditions, the normal reaction of the body is to pour hormones, such as cortisone, and adrenaline, into the blood stream, thus increasing blood pressure, heart rate and breath intake and preparing us for fight or flight. Obviously, this is highly necessary in the appropriate circumstances, but unfortunately we can become unconsciously locked in this condition, even though facing far less demanding situations. For example, pressures from personal relationships, financial worries, fears of redundancy, bottled-up resentment, frustration, niggling anxieties and fears, one or all can add fuel to the Flight-Fight Response, so that we rarely switch off, if at all. The body is consequently forced to produce steroids which can interfere with our protective immune system and the increase in metabolism produced by stress may well use up valuable energy needed for the maintenance of health. All of us produce many thousands of cancer cells daily; under normal conditions, these are efficiently dealt with by the immune system. If the latter becomes impaired, however, the cancer cells may get out of hand. It also followed, of course, that an impaired immune system lays our bodies open to other diseases as well, so it is in the interest of our own present and future well being that we learn to recognize a condition of stress in ourselves which has got out of hand. We then learn to relax into a restful state in which the blood pressure and heart rate drops and the body can recharge, revitalize and resuscitate its immune system. Besides, this is a delightful state and should be seen to be as nourishing for the body as good food and proper breathing. Lack of attention to the fundamental needs of the body may cause more disease than tension itself.

Everyone should learn to relax

Apart from being an effective way of coping positively with stress and disorders it causes, relaxation helps us to avoid unnecessary fatigue and to recover from it more quickly. It gives the body's own natural healing rhythms a chance to function more efficiently. It can raise the threshold of tolerance to pain. It aids personal relationships which can be such a cause of tension, because it is easier to get on with people when you are relaxed and at ease. It also helps us to sleep better and enhances our feeling of well-being.

"Dis-ease": An Inner State

Through relaxation the body is able to resolve the physical tension which can arise from the day to day challenges of living. The real causes of tension, however, lie within ourselves and cannot really be blamed on others. It is our inability to come to terms with situations and conditions in ourselves that leads us to a state of resistance, be it of a forceful nature, or one of apathy. The mind will contrive most wonderfully to justify our own negative attitudes and actions, including the stands we take in our relationships with others. Relaxation of the body alone will not resolve these inner conflicts. We will need to go deeper into the process of training the mind to become positive and one-pointed in bringing about a state of well-being within ourselves.

Meditation

This leads us to Meditation. There are many forms of meditation, but our main motivation in meditating is to heal ourselves in whatever way is appropriate.

In seeking true health, we may need to understand the relationship between body, mind and spirit and it is important to realize what power the mind has in directing thoughts either creatively or destructively. And energy follows thought. The mind can be likened to a conductor of an orchestra. The orchestra can be conducted so that each member gives of his or her best and harmony results, or there can be a lack of coordination and discord. If the latter arises in the orchestra of our bodily, emotional, mental and spiritual needs, then we experience dis-ease in some form. It is our responsibility to see how our own mind directs its thoughts positively towards the well being of the whole.

First of all, let us be quite clear, meditation is not an opting out of life. Rather it enables us to live life more fully – more usefully and more creatively. It enables us to enrich the relationship of body, mind and spirit, through which true healing flows.

The first thing we need to achieve is relaxation. We cannot meditate if we are not relaxed, although we can be relaxed and not meditating. Deepening degrees of relaxation can lead us naturally towards mediation. These are stages on the way. The mind, however, has to be encouraged to become one pointed, alert and poised. It has to be trained to cease from showering us with uninvited thoughts, such as items for the shopping list, or the state or our bank balance! The required state might be likened to a sentry on duty on a moonless night: body relaxed and composed, but senses alert for the slightest indication of noise of an intruder. There is no question of going to sleep!

A Daily Routine

Initially, we could say reaching a meditative state involves four things; we could call them "Four Quiet States". When our health is involved, it is important to try and set aside three periods of relaxation/meditation of 10 to 20 minutes each and every day. It is only as difficult as you yourself make it, though young children add an extra challenge! You can spend 10 or 20 minutes when you awake and again before you go to sleep at night. To begin with the mind finds all sorts of excuses but it responds to firmness, kindness and a sense of humor!

The Four Quiet States

1. A Quiet Environment — a place where you feel "at ease", free from door bells, or telephone. This is **your** special time. There is no need to feel in the least guilty in allowing time to revitalize your body and to link with your innermost resources.

2. A Quiet Body — this means a relaxed body in a comfortable position with a straight spine. Whatever position you adopt, be it lying, sitting, kneeling, or full lotus, if you are too cozy, you run the risk of falling asleep. If so, the relaxation you achieve will be from the body only and even then the body does not necessarily relax fully in sleep. The deepest relaxation is attained when the mind is involved also.

3. A Quiet Receptive Attitude — perhaps most important of all. Don't strive for goals, don't expect anything, rather ALLOW relaxation to happen. Allow the breath to deepen in the abdomen, not in the upper chest. The deepening of the breath in the abdominal region has a steadying, calming effect and draws us into deeper relaxation.

4. A Quiet Mind — "quiet" in the context of being "unbusy", but alert and poised. This may require the repetition of a special word, or mantra to keep the mind focused; quietly concentrating on the ebb and flow of the breath is another method; using a symbol or image which evokes a state of well-being, or the innermost source of all true healing; is yet another.

Whatever method proves most appropriate for us is what matters, thereafter meditation can help us reactivate our powers of healing and find an inner peace which enables us to enjoy life more fully.

— 17 —

CREAM OF CATHAY

Miracles still happen!!

*T*he man walked into the Las Vegas Gym and he was beaming with good reason. The skin cancer that had plagued him for many years had gone completely in three days. He estimated a cost of two thousand dollars spent with dermatologist and other experts all to no avail, yet, just by a crazy fluke he had rid himself of this disease in three days at no cost at all.

He was the fourth person to discover the solution in the past two weeks, so most of us were getting used to hearing about it.

They had all simply discovered what the Indians of South America had known for the past six thousand years. They would boil the bark of a very special tree that grows in their rain forest, and spread the solution on their faces and bodies. The Vikings, that visited them in those far-off days, often took home boatloads of the bark, which proved even more valuable than gold. (From the book, **Killing Cancer,** Vinton Publishing).

Strangely enough, medical science in America has recently found that this bark contains a very powerful antibiotic.

At the same time the Vikings were visiting South America, the Chinese at the ancient city of Xian were treating all skin problems with a herbal solution which was quite powerful. It seldom failed to get results. In America, seven American and Chinese doctors worked together investigating this herb, along with others. They chose to call it the FU-ZHENG therapy and they proved to everyone's satisfaction that these herbs are most powerful. "American Cancer Society 0008-543x83/0701/0070."

Can you imagine the results if these two products mentioned above were combined into a smooth, cool, healing cream?

We did this last year in London, then a scientist came to us with the natural fragrance of rosewater, in use since before the birth of Christ. Cleopatra would bathe in rose water each day. The petals, gathered by virgins dressed in long white robes, would only be picked by the light of the moon. Rosewater was also the most popular fragrance during the life of Christ.

Jason Winters was the first person to mix these astonishing ingredients together into a thick cooling healing cream, with the fragrance of roses on a summer evening.

This skin care cream has already attracted the attention of the cosmetic trade, and also inquiries from the world's largest suntan lotion company who wish to make it the base for all cosmetics and oils.

Mr. Rolpha top cosmetic chemist claims that Cream of Cathay is the ultimate beauty cream for softness, coolness and the look of vibrant health.

Next we added the worlds best astringent from Argentina – called "INORE" so now you can look younger too!!

— 18 —

HEART TROUBLES AND HIGH BLOOD PRESSURE

A common remedy for heart troubles and high blood pressure is cayenne liquid. Within a few moments the blood pressure of most people is back to normal and all pain is gone.

Easily available in Australia, and selling in massive quantities, this natural, harmless "food" is almost impossible to obtain in America. From what we are led to believe, heart problems are the number 1 killer in North America, so I leave it to the reader to draw his own conclusions as to why cayenne liquid is not available to everyone.

In Sydney, New South Wales a man of forty dropped down with extreme heart pains right in the middle of the street. A lady from a nearby house had watched what had taken place and calmly walked out and leaning over the man, placed a pillow under his head. Then she spooned a little cayenne liquid into the man's mouth. Within three minutes the pains had stopped and the man got up and walked away. The policeman on the spot was flabbergasted, the paramedics were upset to learn that their patient had escaped them, and there was talk of charging the helpful lady with practicing medicine without a license, but the case was dropped.

Have you ever seen a car accident in America, where tow trucks, all listening to the police radio band, rush to the spot like vultures, each one trying desperately to hook on to one car or another to insure themselves seventy-five dollars or more? Well, sometimes ambulance drivers remind me of the same thing. In Las Vegas one hospital guarantees that if you take an ambulance to their hospital, and you have to check in, they will pay the ambulance fee. It's almost like paying a finders fee for obtaining an investor in a company.

— 19 —

WHITE SUGAR AND THE REPRODUCTIVE SYSTEM

*I*t wasn't until Peter Hill and his wife Jean moved onto the farm they had purchased that they noticed the ants. There were millions of them, not only in every room of the house but all over the ten acres they owned. The two children were bitten quite often and the bites were both painful and often infected. They tried spraying thoroughly, but after two days the ants were back. Then they called in professional exterminators, but all to no avail. The ants would disappear for two days, then start coming back worse than ever. The situation became intolerable when the children could not go out to play in the yard, and Peter, working the land, would have fresh bites to contend with each night. They appealed to the "Letters to the editor" of their local newspaper and many solutions came in from friends and neighbors, but nothing worked.

One day, however, when things looked their worst, a small booklet was sent to them through the mail. It was written in the Greek language and the sender had been concerned enough to write the English translation under each line. The author said it was guaranteed to work. The solution was to purchase 500 lbs. of white refined sugar, and pour little piles five inches high in every room of the house, and in all covered areas of the land, such as in hollow logs, under boards and anywhere that the piles would not get wet.

In desperation they did this exactly as described in the booklet. They had hundreds of little piles all over their land. In four months there was not an ant to be found, and they have never returned. Now the reader may be excused for being skeptical, for I was also when I read the report. I thought that if you fed the ants, especially with delicious white sugar, the population would increase, not disappear entirely. But I had forgotten one thing. The sugar was delicious, but absolutely non-nutritious, and highly toxic, which over three generations of ants (four months), broke down their health and destroyed their reproductive system so they could not have young. This is exactly what's happening to the human race but on a slower pace because our generations are many years, not weeks as are the ants.

HANNE KRAMB ON SEX

A 73 year old man came to the clinic complaining that he had a forty-two year old wife, but found that it was impossible for him to have sexual intercourse, because of his age.

Hanne gave him acupuncture, and injections of calves liver, pancreas and brain, along with Xian capsules. Within one month the man's wife called the clinic and asked Hanne Kramb if there was something she could give him to slow him down. Evidently it had worked too well. Sadly, nothing can be done for this man. One can only hope that his new found vigor will cool as time goes by.

People visiting the Hanne Kramb clinic at Christmas time are astounded at what they find. Hundreds of gifts start arriving from grateful people all over the world, people that will never forget her, and the help she gave them. I understand from one patient that the gifts fill up four complete rooms.

It seems as though GOD is using people like Hanne

Kramb to spread love, health and happiness to those who have had all hope taken away from them by the so-called orthodox people.

The two products necessary for rejuvenation are Xian capsules and/or Solcosplen tablets, depending upon your condition.

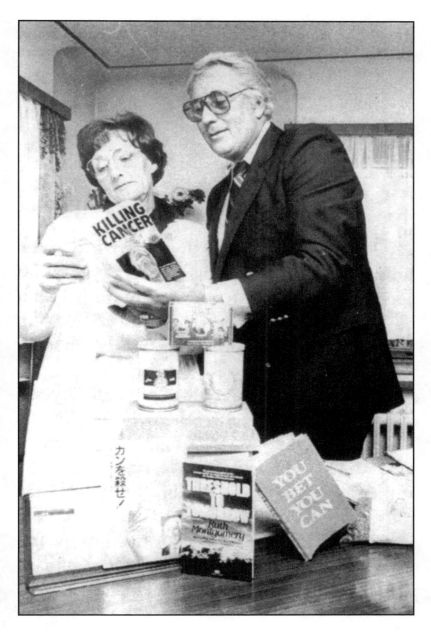

Miracle Lady Hanne Kramb goes over certain points in Jason's book in the German language.

— 21 —

THE MIRACLE LADY OF HONZRATH

*A*72 year old medical doctor arrived at the clinic on a stretcher. He had been to see all his medical friends in a desperate bid for help but they could not help him. They had all told him to go home and prepare to die. He was in fact a hopeless case.

Told constantly that he was after all 72 years old and could expect problems like this, he finally gathered enough strength to sign himself out of the hospital, and, as a last resort, had the ambulance people take him to the Hanne Kramb clinic. Told by his medical doctors to take three tablets each day for his Parkinson's disease, he did, on the day he signed himself out of the hospital take ten of them. His shaking was so very bad that it was almost impossible to work on him.

That man, three months later is back at work, running his own practice again with no shaking and no illness of any kind. The doctor's family has stated publicly that they would never seek help from anyone other than Hanne Kramb again. I arrived in Luxemburg on April the 4th,

1984, to be interviewed by a large magazine and also local newspapers. It was then that I started hearing these remarkable stories everywhere I turned. I decided that I must visit this clinic myself, and arrived just a few days later. It was an hour's drive from the Luxemburg airport, across the border into West Germany. The clinic was located in the beautiful town of Honzrath, and was situated on the top of a tree studded hill.

The atmosphere was just like home, with everyone so friendly and kind. Hanne Kramb had used my Tribalene in her practice for a long time and that certainly was a pleasant surprise to me.

I at once issued her the challenge, "What's the matter with me?" purposely while the media was still there doing my interview. She asked me to look into the end of a magnifying glass while she looked into the other end in order to study my left eye. At once she said that I had kidney damage and a backbone out of alignment especially at my neck.

She was right on both counts. Years before, I had suffered kidney damage while playing soccer, and also, because I "headed" the ball so much I had injured my neck muscles. Doctors had told me that for years, after expensive tests and many questions, yet this lady knew it at once with no questions at all.

The news media took photos of her treating me with acupuncture and a neck adjustment, which took fifteen minutes to correct both situations. She also took another five minutes to correct my constantly draining sinuses. The effect was immediate. She simply opened up the blocked nerves that were causing the problem, and at once the drainage took place in my nose instead of the back of my throat.

DEATH BEGINS IN THE COLON

Important Discussion of Alimentary Toxemia Before the Royal Society of Medicine of Great Britain

*R*ecently, the subject of alimentary toxemia was discussed in London before the Royal Society of Medicine, by fifty-seven of the leading physicians of Great Britain. Among the speakers were eminent surgeons, physicians, and specialists in the various branches of medicine.

Poisons of Alimentary Intestinal Toxemia

The following is a list of the various poisons noted by several speakers: Indol, phenol, cresol, indican, sulphurretted hydrogen, ammonia, histidine, indican, urrobilin, methylmercaptan, tetramerhylendiamin, pentamethy lendiamine, putrescin, cadaverin, neurin, cholin, muscarine, butyric acid, bera-imidazzolethylamine, methylgandinine, ptomarropine, botulin, tyramine, agamatine, tryptophane, sepsin, idolethylamine, sulpher-roglobine.

Of the 36 poisons mentioned above, several are highly active, producing most profound effects, and in very small quantities. In cases of alimentary toxemia some one or several of these poisons is constantly bathing the delicate body cells, and setting up charges which finally result in grave disease.

Symptoms and Diseases Due to Alimentary Toxemia

It should be understood that these findings are not mere theories, but are the results of demonstrations in actual practice by eminent physicians. Of course it is not claimed that alimentary toxemia is the only cause of all the symptoms and diseases named. Although of many it may be the sole or principal cause, some of them are due to other causes as well. In the following summary the various symptoms and disorders mentioned in the discussion in London, to which reference has been made above, are grouped and classified.

THE DIGESTIVE ORGANS

Duodenal ulcer causing partial or complete obstruction of the duodenum; pyloric spasm; pyloric obstruction; distention and dilation of the stomach; gastric ulcer, cancer of the stomach; adhesions of the omentum to the stomach and liver; inflammation of the liver; cancer of the liver.

The muscular wall of the intestine as well as other muscles atrophy, so that the passage of their contents is hindered. The abdominal visceral lose their normal relationship to the spine and to each other, on account of weakening of the abdominal muscles; these displacements are much more marked and serious in women. Other conditions are: Catarrh of the intestines; foul gases and foul smelling stools; colitis; acute enteritis; appendicitis, acute and chronic; adhesions and "kinks" of the intestines; visceroptosis; enlargement of spleen, distended abdomen; tenderness of the abdomen; summer diarrhea of children; inflammation of pancreas; chronic dragging abdominal pains; gastritis; cancer of pancreas; inflammatory changes of gall bladder, cancer of gall bladder; gallstones; degeneration of liver; cirrhosis of liver; infection of the gums, and decay of the teeth; ulcers in the mouth and pharynx.

HEART AND BLOOD VESSELS

Wasting and weakening of the heart muscles; microbic cyanosis from breaking up of blood cells; fatty degeneration of the heart; endocarditis; subnormal blood pressure; enlargement of the heart; the dilitation of the aorta; high blood pressure; arteriosclerosis; permanent dilation of arteries.

Dr. W. Bezley says: "There are a few phases of cardiovascular trouble (disease of heart and blood vessels) with which disorder of some part of the alimentary tract is not causatively associated."

THE NERVOUS SYSTEM

Headaches of various kinds – frontal, occipital, temporal, dull or intense, hemicrania; headache of a character to **lead to a mistaken diagnosis of brain tumor.** Dr. Lane tells of a case where a surgeon had proposed an operation for the removal of a tumor from the frontal lobe of the brain; the difficulty was wholly removed by the exclusion of the colon. Acute neuralgia pains in the legs; neuritis, twitching of the eyes and of muscles of face, arms, legs, etc. Lassitude; irritability;

disturbances of nervous system, varying from simple headaches to absolute collapse; mental and physical depression. Insomnia; troubled sleep, unpleasant dreams; unrefreshing sleep, the patient awakening tired; excessive sleepiness, patient falling asleep in the daytime; shivery sensation across lower spinal region; burning sensations in face, hands, etc.; epileptiform tic; typhoid state; paralysis; chronic fatigue; horror of noises; morbid introspection; perverted moral feelings; melancholia, mania, loss of memory; difficult of mental concentration; imbecility; insanity; delirium, coma.

THE EYES

Degenerative changes in the eye; inflammation of the lens; inflammation of the optic nerve; hardening of the lens; sclerotitis; sclerokeratitis; iritis; iridocyclitis; cataract; recurrent hemorrhage in the retina; eye dull and heavy.

THE SKIN

Formation of wrinkles; thin, inelastic, starchy skin; pigmentations of the skin – yellow, brown, slate-black, blue; muddy complexion; offensive secretion from the skin of flexures; thickening of the skin of the back of the skin – sores and boils; pemphigus; pruritus; herpes; eczema; dermatitis; lupus erythemarosus; acne rosacrea; cold, clammy extremities; dark circles under the eyes; seborrhea; psoriasis; pityriasis; alopecia, lichen; planus; jaundice; "An infinitesimal amount of poison may suffice to cause skin eruption".

MUSCLES AND JOINTS

Degeneration of the muscles; "Muscles waste and become soft and in advanced cases tear easily. In young life the muscular debility produces the deformities which are called dorsal excurvation, or round shoulders, lateral curvature, flat-feet, and knock-knees." Weakness of abdominal muscles causes accumulation of feces in the pelvic colon, which renders evacuation of contents more and more difficult. Prominence of bones; rheumatic pains simulating sciatica and lumbago; various muscular pains; muscular rheumatism; arthritis deformities; synavitis, rickets; arthritis, acute and chronic. Tubercle, and rheumatoid arthritis are the direct result of intestinal intoxication. Dr. Lane says "I do not believe it is possible for either of these diseases to obtain a foothold except in the presence of stasis."

GENITO-URINARY AND REPRODUCTIVE ORGANS

Various displacements, distortion and disease of the uterus; change in the whole forms contour of woman; fibrosis of breast; wasting of breasts; induration of breasts; sub-acute and chronic mastitis; cancer of breast; merritis and endomestritis; infection of bladder especially in women; frequent urination; albumosuria; acute nephritis; moveable kidney; floating kidney. Dr. Lane goes so far as to say: "Autointoxication plays so large a part in the development of disease of the female genito-urinary apparatus, that they may be regarded by the gynecologist as a product of intestinal stasis."

GENERAL DISORDERS AND DISTURBANCES OF NUTRITION

Degeneration of the organs of elimination, especially the liver, kidneys (Bright's disease) and spleen; pernicious anemia; lowered resistance to infection of all kind; premature senile decay; retardation of growth in children, accompanied by mental irritability and muscular fatigue; adenoids, enlarged tonsils; scurvy; enlarged thyroid (goiter); various tumors and thyroid; Raynaud's disease. In those who apparently suffer no harm from constipation during a long series of years there is perhaps, as suggested by Hertz, a partial immunity established. The writer has long believed that such an immunity is sometimes established in the very obstinate constipation which accompanies absolute fasting, because of the cleansing of the tongue and reappearance of appetite which often occurs at the end of the second or third week of the fast, a phenomenon very like that which appears in typhoid fever and other continued fevers. It must not be supposed, however, that even the establishment of so-called immunity insures the body against all injury. The labor of eliminating an enormous amount of virulent toxins, which falls upon the kidneys, damages the renal tissues and produces premature failure of these essential organs. Any process which develops toxins within the body is a menace to the life of the tissues and should be suppressed as far as possible, and as quickly as possible.

The fact that symptoms of poisoning resulting from constipation do not appear at once is no evidence that injury is not done. Dr. William Hunter in the course of the London discussion remarked that the fact that chronic constipation "might exist in certain individuals as an almost permanent condition without apparently causing ill health is due solely to the power and protective action of the liver. It is not any evidence of the comparative harmlessness of constipation per se, but only an evidence that some individuals possess the cecum and the colon of an ox, with the liver of a pig, capable of doing any amount of distoxication." In the face of such an array of evidence backed up by authority of nearly 60 eminent English physicians – and many hundreds of other English, U.S., German and French physicians whose names might be added – it is no longer possible to ignore the importance of alimentary toxemia or autointoxication as a fact in the production of disease. To no other single cause is it possible to attribute one-tenth as many various and widely diverse disorders. **"It may be said that almost every chronic disease known is directly or indirectly due to the influence of bacterial poisons absorbed from the intestine.** The colon may be justly looked upon as a veritable Pandora's box, out of which come more human misery and suffering, mental and moral, as well as physical than from any other source."

The colon is a sewage system, but by neglect and abuse it becomes a cesspool. When it is clean and normal we are well and happy; let it stagnate, and it will distill the poisons of decay, fermentation and putrefaction into the blood, poisoning the brain and nervous system so that we become mentally depressed and irritable; it will poison the heart so that we are weak and listless; poison the lungs so that the breath is foul; poison the digestive organs so that we are distressed and bloated; and poison the blood so that the skin is sallow and unhealthy. In short, every organ of the body is poisoned, and we age prematurely, look and feel old, the joints are stiff and painful, neuritis, dull eyes and a sluggish brain overtake us; the pleasure of living is gone.

The preceding information should impress you with the vital importance of bowel regularity to you and every member of your family.

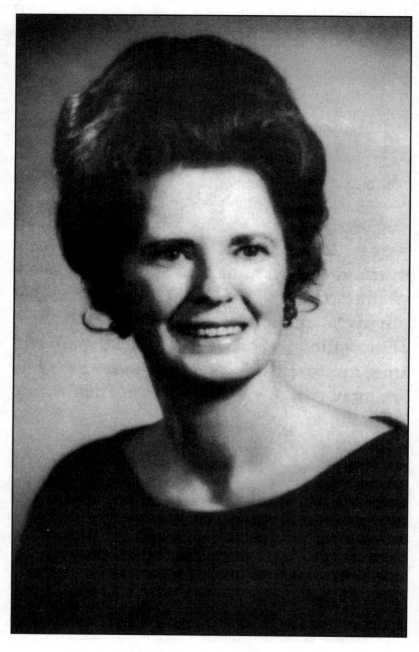

Dr. Vanity Forsyth – Leading Authority on the Colon
Doctor of Chiropractic

— 23 —

THE COLON

When I decided to write about a complete cleanse for body, mind and spirit I fully knew the importance of the colon.

In my search for the right expert in the field for colon therapy the name Dr. Vanity Forsyth came up again and again. I located her in Kingman, Arizona, but only after I had found out the following:

During her life she had always suffered from bowel problems, which resulted in the loss of her colon, long intestine, the rectum and part of the small intestine, surgically.

When it was too late for her, she found the importance of a clean colon and regular bowel movements, and so has devoted her whole life to helping others avoid the tragedy that she endured.

She is now an expert in her field, and where others would have given up on life completely after such an operation, Dr. Forsyth had just started to live and to fight.

Thousands of people have benefited from her knowledge, and people can only suspect what terrible illness and operations they would have had to endure had they not changed their way of life, after talking to this lady.

Dr. Forsyth has been there. She has eaten wrongly, suffered the consequences of a horrible operation. What better person for America to turn to, and of course, people are, by the thousands.

Following is an interview with this most remarkable, attractive lady.

SIGNS THAT YOU NEED THE BOWEL BOUTIQUE

• If you are tired all the time
• If you have to tip the bell boy to help you carry the bags under your eyes
• If your abdomen hangs down over your belt
• If your friends are planning a surprise baby shower for you and you're not pregnant
• If your face is bloated
• If your bowel movements smell so bad, you can't stand to be in the same room with yourself
• If your 24 hour deodorant surrenders in 24 minutes
• If your wife won't kiss you anymore because of your foul breath and draining sinuses
• If your eyes are so bloodshot you have to go to the blood bank to have them drained
• If you weigh in on a public scale and the card comes back, "One at a time please."

• If you tell your husband every night, "Sorry, I have a headache," and you really do

• If you pass wind in the office and your secretary passes out

• If your eyelids hang down over your eyes so far, you look like you're asleep

• If when you take off your socks, the dog leaves the room

• If your body odor would put a skunk to shame

• If every time you belch, it kicks on the air conditioner

DO YOU RECOMMEND LAXATIVES?

No, not as a routine thing. Do you realize there are more than 40,000 laxatives used in America today, so that should give you an idea what kind of shape the country is in.

I would recommend them only under certain circumstances. But not as a habit, unless there is no other way. The catch is, most people THINK there is no other way, that is why this bowel cleaning program may be the answer to their prayers. Laxatives are recommended when you begin the bowel cleaning program for the first 3 days only. One lady had to take laxatives for 25 years and is completely dependent on them. Her bowels **will not move** at all without 6 strong laxatives every night. I even recommended Dr. Christopher's Nature-lax 2 which tones and strengthens, cleanses and provides some laxative effect. It didn't help moving the bowel. Her bowel is damaged to the point, I fear, that she will never be able to do without laxatives. Even if laxatives were safe, they still wouldn't remove those deposits that have been building and hardening in you for years.

WHAT MAKES PEOPLE CONSTIPATED?

There are two major reasons for this: One — When the food you eat is not ALL expelled within a day or two, this is constipation, whether you realize it or not. This leads to too long retention of feces, causing it to harden and dry out as too much moisture is reabsorbed from the colon, clogging and irritating the nerve endings in the bowel lining. Two — Eating the wrong foods: a) A diet high in mucous forming foods, such as sugars, dairy products, meat, eggs, processed highly refined foods, white flour, cooked foods and not enough raw. b) A diet low in fiber. High fibrous foods include raw fruits and vegetables, steamed or baked fruits and vegetables, whole grains, beans, peas, lentils, etc. c) Not drinking enough plain, pure water.

Medications – antibiotics are famous for wiping out the good guys in the bowel (the favorable intestinal flora, leaving it wide open for the bad buys, such as harmful bacteria and virus to move in. According to Dr. John Harvey Kellogg the ratio should be about 85% acidophilis and 15% bacillus coli (bad guys). These bad guys thrive on undigested protein (mostly meat) and are gas producers. This ratio is usually reversed in most people and the bad guys outnumber the good guys 85% - 15%.

The Bible states: "Why do you take into your body, that which your body has no need."

One autopsy revealed a colon to be 9" in diameter with a passage through it no larger than a pencil! The rest was caked up layer upon layer of encrusted fecal material. This accumulation can have the consistency of truck tire rubber. It's hard and black. Another autopsy revealed a stagnant colon to weigh in at an incredible 40 pounds! Imagine carrying around all that morbid accumulated waste.

When the bowel is dirty, it can harbor an amazing variety of very harmful bacteria and parasites. It's interesting to note that worms outrank cancer as man's deadliest enemy on a world-wide basis! It is estimated that 200 million people are infected by these intestinal parasites.

These worms range in size from microscopic single-celled animals to 2-ft. long tapeworms! These parasites kill more people annually than does cancer. One in four people in the world today are infected by roundworms. The U.S. is not immune to these parasites, as the number of cases has increased in the past few years.

It is my opinion that more people than this have parasites. A lot of them have never been diagnosed properly. I might add, it could be as high as 80%. I was one of them. It can happen to you.

WHAT SIZE SHOULD THE PROPER STOOL BE?

"When your colon is healthy, you will have 2 well formed bowel movements a day. Every morning, you'll have a huge movement which should altogether be 2-4 feet long. Later on in the day you'll have another movement, which will be about one half the size of the first. These stools should be expelled effortlessly – within seconds after you sit down." — V.E. Irons, Healthview Newsletter #10.

Obviously if the stools are long and size of a pencil or look like rabbit pellets, or if they are short and hard and if you pass mucous, blood or half-digested food, this is indicative of poor bowel function.

SHOULD NORMAL STOOL BE THE SAME COLOR?

Yes, the color should generally be about the same – brown, this may vary temporarily depending on what you eat. e.g., beets or spinach will affect the color, but if it is grey or yellow, something is wrong.

DO MANY PEOPLE SUFFER FROM A POOR COLON?

About 95% of the population. The other 5% has either been on a perfect diet since birth or live in the Himalayas.

It is estimated that over 75 million Americans suffer from bowel problems. The second leading cause of death in the cancer field is cancer of the bowel, more than 100,000 people a year die from colon cancer.

Colitis and diverticulitis affect probably over two and a half million people.There are approximately 125,000 people who undergo a radical colostomy or ilestomy per year. I was one of them.

Even the American Cancer Society state, "Evidence in recent years suggests that most bowel cancer is caused by environmental agents. Some scientists believe that a diet high in beef and/or low in fiber is the cause."

DOCTORS TELL MANY PEOPLE THAT ONE BOWEL MOVEMENT EVERY TWO DAYS IS FINE. WHAT DO YOU THINK?

I think it is absolutely ridiculous. I've even known some

doctors to say that even once a week may be normal for you. Do they also think it is "normal" to have a bowel lined with black hardened mucous since I'm sure most everyone undergoing surgery or autopsies has it, so it must be normal.

Years ago, the famous Dr. Harvey Kellogg of Battle Creek, Michigan said: "Of the 22,000 operations I have personally performed, I have never found a single normal colon." If Dr. Kellogg made this comment around 1900 just imagine how much worse the situation is today.

DO YOU BELIEVE THAT COLON PROBLEMS CAUSE OTHER ILLNESSES?

Very definitely yes. I have personally seen the following conditions either clear up completely or be greatly improved as soon as the person cleansed their bowel: headaches; sciatic; stiff neck; arthritis; psoriasis; high blood pressure; swollen tonsils; pneumonia, flu and colds; allergies; sinus; skin eruptions; eye problems; constipation; paralyzed bowel; chronic fatigue; liver spots on head and face; leg cramps; frequent urination; chronic pain inside and more. We can't cure old age, but we can postpone it for a while. "There is really no incurable disease, only incurable people."

— Dr. John Christopher

WHAT CAUSES A LAZY COLON AND BOWEL?

The bowel soon becomes overburdened with accumulated toxic wastes and poisons. It's unable to throw off these poisons.

Let's visualize the following scenario: You have a perfect bowel, you are on a perfect diet. Once in a while you ingest something that is harmful (remember, anything that is not a food, the body treats as a poison). In order to protect itself, the body causes mucous to be formed in the colon long before the harmful food or substance reaches there. The substance reaches the colon 18 hours later (remember, you have a perfect colon and things move along right on schedule). The mucous has been prepared by the body and is lining the colon so you won't absorb the poison when it gets there, so it literally coats the poison. Then later it breaks down and will be discharged from the colon with no harmful effect. Well, you got away with it that time. Nature's protective mechanism functioned properly. So you do it more often.

Four times today, you ingested mucous forming foods. Most of which is also low fiber. The mucous is secreted four times today to protect you against what you just ate and drank, and smoked. So, you do this every day of your life but every day you TRY to eat something raw, on apple or orange or salad (maybe) this helps. but 85-90% of everything you eat is going to cause mucous to be formed. THE MUCOUS LINING IN THE BOWEL THICKENS.

Nature's protective mechanism, which was designed for occasional use only, is being forced to work continuously day after day, year after year, with no rest and no chance to eliminate the mucous which is being laid down faster than it can be eliminated. Layer piles upon layer, like the rings of a tree.

IS A HEAVY BRAN DIET
GOOD FOR YOU?

You can't expect to erase the abuses of a lifetime by taking a couple tablespoons of bran. Heavy doses of bran CAN be dangerous for a lot of people. Bran can only propel the new daily fecal matter thru the already clogged colon. It will not sweep out the hardened encrusted mucous and hard fecal impactions, nor will any other roughage. If you had started out as a child eating diets high in roughage and fiber, you wouldn't be in this shape today and large doses of bran would be fine.

I realize that some people are in such bad shape they are grateful for any small measure of relief bran can afford. They tell me – I have to have bran every morning or I can't go at all. (How much more relief would they get if they cleaned out their entire colon of the putrid decaying material!!!!) If you get relief from bran, don't stop using it, but be careful if the colon is looped, bent , twisted, etc., bran can get stuck in the loose mucous (which can be in there by the quarts,) and clog you up completely. The psyllium seed powder (intestinal cleanser) is 100 times better than bran. It is non-irritating and absorbs huge quantities of water, softens and lubricates.

DO HEMORRHOIDS HAVE ANYTHING TO DO WITH CONSTIPATION?

That would be the major contributing factor. I feel that the pressure from a backed up distended colon and the straining from constipation (causes the blood vessels to stretch in the lower part of the colon and rectum. It then becomes enlarged, fills with blood, gets sore and itches), along with loss of muscle tone, would be the main cause.

YOU MENTION A SEVEN DAY FAST. ISN'T ANOTHER WAY TO BECOME HEALTHY WITH FASTING?

First of all, I would like to clarify this. True fasting means the abstinence from any type of food or drink, except water. This program is not a true fast. Actually I prefer to call this a 7-day cleanse. Of course during the 7-day cleanse, you are drinking only liquids. Some juice, as well as water, JWT, and some vegetable broth. Absolutely no solid food.

The following is the program I recommend:
• The 7-day bowel cleansing program done every 7-8 weeks, using the Jason Winter's Tea.

• Continuation of use of intestinal cleanser once or twice a day.

• This followed by as perfect a diet as you can manage. The complete mucous free diet, as much raw food as possible.

• Drink lots of pure water and exercise.

WOULD YOU EXPLAIN YOUR COMPLETE PROGRAM IN ITS ENTIRETY?

This cleanse can be done every 2 months for a year or more, or however long it takes to cleanse the bowel completely. I suggest at least twice a year as a maintenance program. After the initial year or year and a half. Not only does this cleanse the bowel and tissues of the body, but gives the glands and organs a rest.

EAT NO SOLID FOOD for the full 7 days. Drink only filtered juices: apple, orange, grapefruit, grape, pineapple, carrot, etc. Do not drink unfiltered (whole fruit) juices; such as tomato, V-8, prune, apricot nectar, etc. JW Sprinkle is excellent. Broth from vegetable soup, made from fresh vegetables. I allow my patients to have a cup or two of hot broth made from powdered raw vegetables and barley.

The night before you start the cleanse:
HERBAL laxative tablets (included with the powder).
The second night, take one and the third night take one.
If desired for stubborn cases, inject (using an infant rectal
syringe) 1 cup of olive oil into rectum. Try to retain this
until morning (massage the bowel gently).

Every day for the full 7 days take:
5 times per day – 3 hrs. apart; (four weights over 150 lbs.)
4 times per day – 3 hrs. apart (for weights under 150 lbs.)

1. Pour about 10-12 oz. of water and juice into pint
jar or blender and:

2. Add 1 tablespoon of clay water (Bentonite, the
intestinal detoxificant)

3. Add last 1 heaping teaspoon of the intestinal
cleanser (Jason Winters colon cleanser)

4. Put cover on and shake violently 12-15 seconds or
blend for a few seconds only (just enough to dissolve)

5. Drink quickly, as it gels fast. Follow with drink of
water, if desired. If it gels too much before you drink it,
don't eat it with a spoon. Add more liquid to thin it down.

**One and a half hours after taking the above
combination take:**
6 Springreen tablets, or Green Life (same thing) –
these are essential.

1 Wheat Germ Oil Capsule

2 Vitamin C Tablets (100mg.)

Take this combination **four** times per day, in between
doses of the cleanse.

At the end of the first day take a coffee enema or home

colonic on the home enema or colonic board. The home boards are highly recommended. They are much more effective and easier than an ordinary enema. Then each morning and evening take an enema.

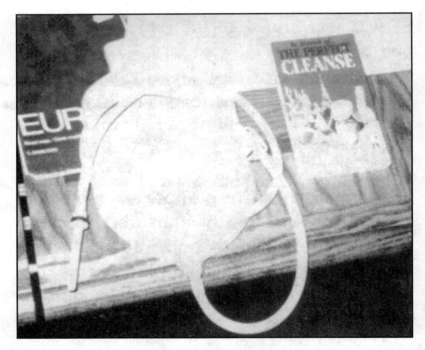

THE ENEMA

This is how to take a coffee enema:

Take one or more enemas daily for the 7-day program and the first day off and follow up for a while 2-3 times a week. Take more if you get a toxic reaction from the cleanse.

Use 4-6 tablespoons of ground coffee (not instant) to 2 quarts water. Simmer 15-20 minutes. Cool to lukewarm.

Do not have water bag hanging too high (about 2 feet above rectum) to prevent too much pressure.

Those of you who have already been taking coffee enemas, perhaps for years, have been instructed to do the following: Lie on side, let in coffee slowly while you draw in a deep breath. Then lie there and retain coffee for 15 minutes, then expel. The purpose of this method is to enable the caffeine to be absorbed through the hemorrhoidal veins and into the portal vein and into the liver. This stimulates the bile ducts to produce bile, causing the detoxification of the liver by causing it to dump accumulated poisons. This is an excellent method for detoxification of the liver. This will pull out a toxic reaction in minutes. Just letting in the coffee and retaining it, will stimulate the bowel walls, and the bowel will rid itself of some of the putrid matter. But without the massaging, you cannot totally accomplish this.

AFTER THE SEVENTH DAY OF CLEANSE

Continue to take the intestinal powder and clay water morning and night until two natural bowel movements a day are established. These products are not laxatives, they are not habit forming. The powder furnishes a fiber that absorbs large quantities of water, but is slippery, soft and very bulky (much more fiber than bran), and is non-irritating. DO NOT STOP TAKING EVERYTHING THE MINUTE THE 7-DAY CLEANSE IS OVER. It may take years to establish normal bowel habits. Just be sure not to take this combination too close to meals, so you won't interfere with food absorption.

Continue to take the Springreen or Greenlife tablets if

desired. The juices from the grasses of grains, is highly nutritious.

To break the fast: On the first day after the cleanse is over, it is imperative you eat only small amounts of raw fruits and vegetables. Do not eat cooked food or junk food, or you may get sick. I know this from experience. Take the supplements.

Second day after the cleanse: Add steamed or baked vegetables, soft boiled eggs (very soft). No bread or dairy products. Use raw veggies and fruit.

Resume normal eating, eliminating sugar, refined flour (white), artificial color, processed foods, junk food.

Drink lots of pure water (between meals).

Continue taking an enema or colonic 1-3 times a week, until bowels become normal. Do not allow stools to become hard or tight. Then take colonics less often.

ACIDOPHILUS – Take a good quality lactobacillus acidophilus after the cleanse to re-establish the intestinal flora washed out by the coffee enemas.

Put a colander in the toilet bowel to catch the mucous accumulations. Most fecal matter will wash through, leaving the accumulations. Then you can see for yourself.

DESCRIPTION OF PRODUCTS

USE ONLY JASON WINTERS COLON CLEANSER (Psyllium Seed, plus husks) a powder that when added to a large amount of water, swells up and becomes mucilaginous, soft and slippery, attaches itself to the mucous lining of the colon, softening and loosening up the hardened encrustations and fecal matter. THIS POWDER IS AN ABSOLUTE NECESSITY FOR THE SUCCESS OF THIS PROGRAM.

INTESTINAL DETOXIFICANT (Bentonite, a clay suspended in water), can absorb 90 times it's weight in toxins from the intestinal tract. An infinitesimal molecule that can literally smother the germ. The active ingredient is Montmorillonite. It's effect is physical rather than chemical.

GREENLIFE OR SPRINGREEN TABLETS: Dried extracted juice of young grains: barley, oats, wheat and rye, raised on soil not sprayed or chemically fertilized. Rich source of vitamins, minerals and enzymes.

COFFEE: Two-fold purpose. 1) Stimulate bowel wall and peristalsis. 2) Stimulating bile production in liver, therefore detoxifying it.

BEET TABLETS: Taken after the 7-day cleanse to have a slight laxative effect and cleanse the liver.

If you have a special health problem, it might be advisable to consult a colon therapist.

ARE COFFEE ENEMAS HABIT FORMING?

At the risk of being facetious, if you drink coffee anyway, what difference does it make?

I certainly would never recommend that anyone drink coffee. So for those of you who object to coffee, don't use it, but don't let that keep you from going on the program.

Use lemon juice, apple cider vinegar, bentonite, epsom salts, or an herb of your choice. Some use chapparell or black walnut.

I've seen coffee irrigations on the board, relieve toxic headache, feverishness, grogginess, leg cramps, aches and pains, etc. or even convulsions (from toxins) in just minutes.

SO WOULD YOU SUGGEST THAT ANYONE ON THE JASON WINTERS PROGRAM OR ANY OTHER HEALTH PROGRAM DO THE SEVEN DAY CLEANSE AS WELL?

Yes, I certainly would. If they have never cleansed their bowel thoroughly I feel they are missing the boat and that they will never be completely healthy until they do this.

I feel this 7-day cleansing program is extremely compatible with Jason Winter's program. For the simple reason, that according to the way I understand it, Jason, is that your program entails a cleansing of the body, with the use of the JW Tribalene, which is also a blood purifier. Therefore, cleaning out a lot of toxins and poisons and rebuilding the body and giving it more strength and endurance. The bowel cleanse can speed up the detoxification process, and more rapidly eliminate the toxins as they are being released. Then after the cleanse, the Tribalene would be absorbed better alone with the other nutrients. Also I find the Tribalene gives you strength and helps sustain you while on the cleanse. You can't just cleanse all the time, you have to rebuild the body.

Dr. John Christopher states that we only absorb

about $\frac{1}{10}^{th}$ of what we eat because of all the mucous buildup, etc. in the colon. After we cleanse the bowel we only require about $\frac{1}{3}$ the food we did previously (he means natural food). But is it any wonder why people are eating all the time, snacking on junk food, etc. They are not absorbing their nutrients and are constantly hungry in the body's attempt to get more nutrition. They are literally starving to death, while consuming too many calories and becoming overweight.

People that have diverticulitis or diverticulosis, or stomach irritation, etc. might not want to change their diet too rapidly and suddenly launch into a high fiber diet, as it might be too harsh to start with. So ease into that a little bit slowly. If you can't eat your salads, drink your salads in the form of raw juice.

DEAD FOOD: If it won't spoil, it's probably dead.

DAIRY PRODUCTS: If possible avoid them. They are all very mucous forming food. They are one of the main causes of allergies, in my opinion, as well as the fact you have a dirty bowel. I've seen people go off sugar and dairy products and sometimes in a few days their allergies are completely gone.

Dr. William A. Ellis of Arlington, Texas, who has researched milk for 42 years claims that the milk protein, casein, is very indigestible to humans, especially infants. Also he claims it has the ability to neutralize hydrochloric acid. Milk and cheese generate a lot of mucous in the bowel and respiratory tracts. Milk can cause constipation as well as diarrhea. According to the Nevada Clinic of Preventative Medicine, (a group of medical doctors that practice homeopathic medicine) in Las Vegas almost 100%

of all patients going through the clinic are allergic to milk. "All books on allergies I've ever studied state that milk and milk products are number one on the list of allergens. A question commonly asked me is, won't you get a calcium deficiency if you don't drink milk? Dr. Ellis stated, "The calcium in cow's milk does not metabolize properly whereas the calcium in mother's milk does. Thousands and thousands of blood tests I've conducted show that people who drink 3 or 4 glasses of milk a day invariably had the lowest levels of blood calcium. Two proteins present in cheese has been known to quite often cause headaches, Tyramine and others.

DON'T DRINK LIQUIDS WITH YOUR MEALS — they dilute the digestive juices down. Drink a nice big drink of whatever you want about 30 minutes before eating. If you are eating the wrong kind of food, that is dry and has to be washed down with a lot of liquid, then that is food to avoid. Natural and raw foods don't cause you to be thirsty with your meals.

CASE HISTORIES

These are the usual type of results:

1. Man in early 40's. Badly bloated, abdomen distended, overweight (mostly from bowel and water retention). Not feeling well, joints in hands aching like arthritis. Hands badly bloated. Could barely hold a pencil to write his name. On the 4th day, he could feel the fluid running out of his fingers. Got out a lot of putrid matter, etc. After 7 days his bloating was completely gone, could write his name, joints don't ache, face looked great. He lost about 15 pounds. Looked very trim.

— J.M. - Kingman, AZ

2. Early 40's. Bloated, chronic shoulder pain, distended abdomen, face, puffy, constipation, high blood pressure, overweight.

After cleanse: bloating gone, lost about 15 pounds; but looked like he had lost 50 because of the bloating. Feeling much better. Blood pressure better. Shoulder pain much improved. Face looked more glowing.

— Mr. C. - Kingman, AZ
— Mr. S. D. - Texas

3. Headaches of 20 years duration gone. Constipation improved. — J.S. - Kingman, AZ

4. Psoriasis on hands – after starting cleanse, psoriasis started to come out of her tissues in arms. Spread over her entire arm area, bilaterally, then went away.

End of Interview

I thought that my colon was in fantastic shape. Dr. Forsyth however laughed at me when I said this. She said that she could prove to me that I needed a cleanse and if I undertook this, I would be amazed at what I passed.

I decided to take her up on it. I would go for seven days without eating and I would do the cleanse exactly as she suggested.

The first two days I was hungry, but taking a half pint of juice (grape) and half a pint of water with the tablespoonful of bentonite and one teaspoonful of the colon cleanser five times each day, stopped me from becoming too uncomfortable.

On the third day I went to the bathroom five times and each time the bowel movement was bigger than I usually had while not on the cleanse. I could not understand where all this "black stuff" was coming from.

When I started on the cleanse I weighed about 250 lbs. The third day I weighed 246. The fourth day of the fast I started passing green mucous, about a half gallon of it. I then weighed 241. I called Dr. Forsyth and asked if this was alright. She could hear the concern in my voice, and when she told me it happens to almost everyone, I felt quite relieved.

The fifth day of not eating, I went to the bathroom five times. Still green mucous now mixed with black hard stuff. Weight at this time 237 lbs.

The sixth day I was not hungry at all. I had three bowel movements this time all hard black fecal matter. Weight 234 lbs. I felt great and was able to get into the clothes that had been placed in the back of my closet because my waist had grown from a 40" to a 46".

On the seventh and last day of the fast I had one bowel movement and passed something four feet long. Once again a panicky call to Dr. Forsyth. She explained that this hardened mucous had been lining my colon for years and I was lucky to be rid of it.

Seventh day 230 lbs., skin great, healthy look, clear eyes, and a determination to do this at least once a year from now on.

Take special note of the fact that if anyone ever gets up off their seats and determines to try something to make them healthier or will give them a better way of life, people gather around to try to talk you out of it.

Listen to me when I say that if they think it's alright to walk around with all that rotting fecal matter, green putrid mucous, bloated stomach, gas indigestion and bad breath, let them go ahead, but don't let them talk you out or your conviction.

I am very proud of one young lady who works at a hair dressing salon in Las Vegas. She went on the seven day fast and cleanse and every day her workmates without exception, tried to talk her into giving it up. Suddenly they all became experts on the subject of fasting and of how bad it is for a person. They forgot how many times in the Bible it tells people to fast.

The world is like that though. People have the urge to talk someone out of something that they can't do themselves, (or think that they can't).

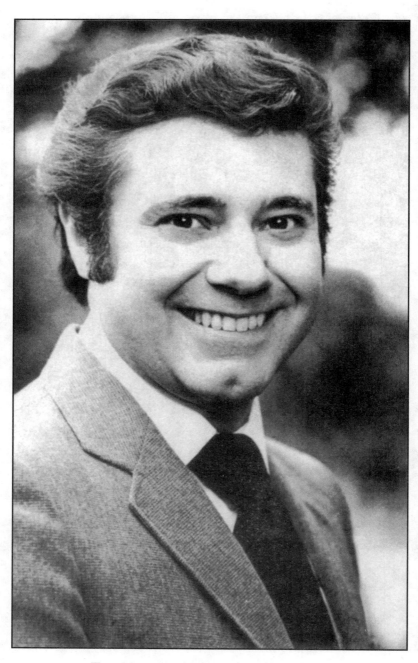

Tony Moscato today, now in Perfect Health.

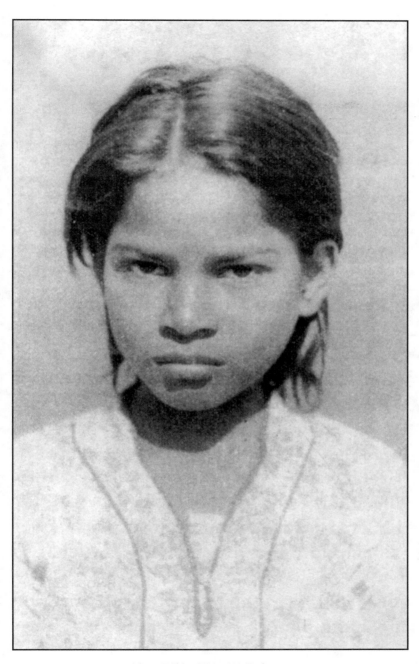

Aleya Bibi - Nassau, Bahamas

— 24 —

AN EVENING WITH TONY MOSCATO

We were staying at the Sheraton British Colonial Hotel in Nassau Bahamas, and were very busy. Our friends from Canada, America and England had all checked into the hotel in order to help us fill the orders for the book, "Killing Cancer".

I had never imagined the popularity and strength of a health magazine known as the "Healthview Newsletter" published in Charlottesville. But they had just published a great story about my beating terminal cancer, and we were receiving around five thousand orders each day.

We took over the board room of that hotel and hired almost every unemployed person that we could find to help us. What a wonderful time that was. Bay Street in Nassau is very popular, with good restaurants and banks, but over the hill is another matter, for this is where the 'ordinary' people live. Most of the huts are just made of wood with no running water or inside toilets. A complete contrast to the tourist section.

A mother came to see me, saying that her daughter, Aleya Bibi had cancer of the face and did not have long to live. She asked me to come with her, over the hill, and to see her daughter. I hesitated to do this for I am no doctor, so am definitely not allowed to heal anyone. That's the law. Her tears overcame me and at last we walked over to the terrible dirty shack she called home. The young girl was in an awful condition, so bad was she that I drew away, which upset me for I was usually overcome with compassion and would hug cancer victims. But this time I drew away with dread. I wanted to run, to escape, for this little girl had the exact same cancer that I had previously had, and in the same place. I quickly told the mother what I would do, if the little girl were mine, and left the shed, and that familiar smell of death that I had last smelled in the cobalt radiation room in America. I was ashamed, but still I fled. Soon after, I left the Bahamas and found myself on a book promotion tour of North America. This was a chance to visit my son in Las Vegas, so I welcomed the opportunity. That is when I first heard of Tony Moscato.

He was handsome, slim and sounded just like Mario Lanza. He would travel California on singing engagements, and would stride onto the stage with confidence and calmness. One day his face started to swell and to ache. It got worse and worse, until the swelling was so large it was affecting his eyes. He went through a biopsy operation, and in May of 1983 returned to his own office, turned on the telephone answering machine to hear the statement, "This is Doctor Ward. The tests show its malignant. It's cancer! Lympho Sarcoma of the Immunoblastic variety." Finding that traditional methods held out no hope for him, he decided to go the alternative therapy route.

He started reading books by the dozens, and found, to his dismay that there were dozens of alternatives, each one stating that it was the very best one, but he was fighting against time, and he didn't have much money. I quote from Tony Moscato's own newsletter:

"Which one to choose? They all seemed to say the same thing: No meat, fish or fowl. No cigarettes. No alcohol. No caffeine. No processed foods. No salt. No sugar. No dairy products. No fried foods. No canned foods. No junk food. No fast food, ONLY LIVE, HEALTHY FOODS to be ingested, and enemas, implants and colonics to cleanse the bowels.

I had stopped smoking a year-and-a-half ago after smoking for 28 years — so that was no problem. Consumption of alcohol was not a part of my life, except when forced to socially accept a drink. Caffeine was another story. I was consuming caffeine not only through coffee, but soft drinks as well. Sodas are very high in sodium.

Although I tried to maintain a balance with health foods at home, I used to indulge, while out, in junk fast-food for a quick pick-me-up.

Every night I had my pint of Haagen-Daz ice cream to fall asleep. My food was not only soft to chew, but very sweet to the taste. On the weekends I loved my omelettes cooked in oodles of creamery butter and topped off with homemade jellies and jams.

With the ominous decree that I had contacted cancer, gone was the stress and depression I had been experiencing. No longer did I have to worry about the house selling or my singing act being booked or making a success with Herbalife products or even marketing my Moscato greeting cards.

All those things were no longer valid in my life. I was benched by the Great Big Manager in the sky and place on the temporarily disabled list. Just like other players in the big leagues of sports, you can't play in the game until you can heal your injuries sufficiently to either carry the ball or at least attempt to carry the ball.

The alternative I chose was WHEAT GRASS THERAPY ... because of the following reasons:

Low-cost, do-it-yourself program

Three week length of time

All raw, living foods

Enemas and implants

Non-toxic drugless regime

No vitamin or mineral pills to take

No injections

Need no helper to do the program

Closest to nature

After four weeks of my own self-induced Raw Foodism program, plus three weeks of the Wheat Grass Juice and Implant Therapy, my cancer cells were adjudged dead. My tumor was down but still evident.

At this point, I immediately transferred to a Macrobiotic diet for balance. My Yin and Yang forces were out of balance and my next priority was to balance my Yin and Yang! The gentleman who suggested this diet was my radionics practitioner. Curiously though, in seven weeks my tumor had almost trebled in size and I was scared to death, confused and in pain twenty-four hours a day. I lived like a dead man – wanting literally to die and get it all over with. I kept asking the Universe to be taken away from all this. I was losing all hope of ever healing this growth that kept growing and putting incredible pressure on my face. The pain was unbearable!

A month previous to all this sad state of affairs, a psychic friend, Crystal Sterling, had told me my healing would come through Jason Winters. I had feebly made an unsuccessful attempt to contact him.

Well, after spending two and one-half hours with an orthomolecular doctor who I believed would help me and relieve me of my pain and pressure, his total negative reactions made me go within myself (my last refuge).

I met a couple, Richard and Ina Wagner, at lunch that day who had spoken personally to Jason Winters and they told me how to reach him in Las Vegas. That evening I called and left a message on their message unit to call me back collect. Jan, his wife, called me the very next morning, Thursday, and on Friday noon she was at the Los Angeles airport delivering the Jason Winters' tea and his book, "Killing Cancer." (As quick as that – the Universe does move quickly when we get out of its way.)

On Monday morning, Jason Winters called me and said, "In six weeks that poison will be out of your face – you have nothing to worry about! All you have to do is drink six glasses of carrot juice daily, eat twenty raw unblanched almonds daily, take six Tribalene capsules and have two coffee enemas each day.

Ladies and gentlemen, within three weeks the poison on my face was gone. That was a miracle! The result of my faith in deciding to listen to my small, soft-speaking voice and, of course, following the nutritional program without deviation. The Universe had answered my prayers.

What an incredibly natural and simple program. How much time had I spent trying all those difficult, demanding and rigidly restrictive diets. In the seemingly interminable search to find my healing – the money that I had worked so hard to save was all spent: the herbalists, accupuncturists, accupressurists, chiropractors, dentists, oral surgeons, ear, nose and throat specialists, oncologists and the never-ending X-rays.

As I now look back over the whole situation, I thank God that I was given the chance of beginning again ... *getting cancer was the greatest thing that ever happened to me!* And I thank Dr. Ward for being the one who diagnosed it for me because, if it were anything less, I would have proceeded on my merry ole way – not changing my life – just skirting the true issues of life and living.

CHANGE is the "open sesame" – the doorkey to every room in God's mansion.

CHANGE is the key word – a person's intimate involvement with the capacity to change is the answer to the question.

WE ARE WHAT WE THINK WE ARE."

Tony Moscato is back singing now, as handsome as he ever was, but an awful lot smarter. He tells his story on radio and TV, giving hope to others. He has written a book called appropriately "You Bet You Can" and it is very interesting reading, whether you have cancer or not.

And oh yes, by the way, if you were wondering about the fate of the little girl, Aleya Bibi, she is now seventeen years of age and very pretty. She is working as a waitress in a cafe on the Bay street.

The reader may well wonder why I put Tony and Aleya in the same chapter. Well, it was the same information that helped Aleya and Tony.

And both are determined to change the world, that the simple truth must not be hidden, that faith can heal, faith can save, and faith if necessary, can move mountains.

Their healing came from faith, a change of mind, a cleansing of the body and nutrition.

Please read chapter 27.

— 25 —

FEAR

*F*rom what I understand, many readers of my books are atheists, agnostics and so on. It is my job to get a message across to these people without them seeing the word, GOD, and quickly turning the page. To those I ask you to please read this short passage which I think will possibly change your life.

It was by no accident that GOD said that we must have faith, for it means far more than the average person thinks it does. You see, faith is the opposite of doubt, so if you do not have faith then you have doubt.

You can no longer rely on anything, because doubt prevails subconsciously in everything you do. Now constant doubt causes worry — a worry causes stress — and stress causes illness and death.

Where there is faith there is no fear, where doubt prevails there is always fear. This is a proven, undisputable fact, proven by the great thinkers of the world, and also proven in my own life.

Fear is the cause of all our problems. It is what causes a good looking teenager to smoke pot, or to stick a needled full of cocaine into his veins. Peer pressure and the fear of not belonging, of not being accepted.

We fear because we doubt and we doubt because we do not have faith enough.

Fear causes stress and we now know that stress destroys the body and mind, resulting in most serious illnesses of today. I have found that people who have an unnatural fear of cancer, get cancer. You see, without faith we are nothing. Without faith in ourselves, our fellow man, our GOD, we become full of despair, suffer from great depression, and can't see any reason to carry on.

If you would rid yourself of fear, stress and illness then you must have faith. If you say that you cannot have faith then it is simply that you have not understood what you have heard and read in the past. Start your own research into religion. Suddenly you will realize that all of this could not have possibly happened by accident. It would take all the genius of the world to make one human hair, then they would fail. Don't listen to atheists who say there is no GOD, for I can tell you first hand that there are no atheists in the front line, nor are there any in the terminal cancer ward.

After a lifetime of fighting GOD, it took me about fifteen seconds to become a Christian, right after the doctor looked at me and said "YOU have terminal cancer, I am going to remove your tongue, jaw bone, tonsils and the inside of your throat, and you will still die in three months."

Suddenly I started talking to GOD, without hesitation, and now I am well, with no operation, no disfigurement, just abundant health.

And so, the lack of faith is tied directly to fear, then stress, then illness. Have faith and you won't fear your peers, you won't need to be an alcoholic, you won't need to be psychotic, or neurotic, you won't have to be up tight all the time, trying to prove yourself everyday. At last you can relax and start doing a better job of living.

What else can I say about fear except that it is at the bottom of all man's problems today. The natural fear that stops you from standing in the middle of the highway is good fear, it protects you, but the constant fear of life, disease, losing your job, your spouse, your manhood is unhealthy and will eventually lead you to the grave.

Over the last ten years, more and more men are complaining of losing their manhood, because they associate with the so-called "liberated woman," who is so dominant and demanding that men are frightened that they won't measure up to this type of woman. Then and there a doubt is formed in the man's mind, and he can't perform. These men are rushing to doctors and psychiatrists offices by the thousands, because they feel that they are not real men any more. Thereby, the liberated woman is ruining things for herself. She has fought against being treated decently, and now people are frightened to open a door for her, or to call her Miss instead of MS or to treat her like a lady.

Today they ask the man to dance, they ask the man to bed, and they scare him to death, and don't let these macho men fool you. Having to perform every night for dominant women eventually causes a breakdown of confidence, the emotions, and brings on great fear. Fear eventually causes illness. And so, as explained in another chapter, the very thing these liberated women are after is being deprived them. Cause and effect. The sad, distressed faces to be seen at any singles bar show that this is not the way. They are all sitting there through fear. Fear of being alone, of not being loved, of not having sex. Faith eliminated all of these doubts and all of these unhealthy activities.

Faith will bring confidence, wisdom, happiness and vibrant health.

CHARLES HEARS OF CANCER DIET

C ANCER patients told Prince Charles how a vegetarian diet and meditation helped them "control" their illness.

They told him of their experiences when he opened the £300,00 controversial Cancer Help Center in Bristol.

Earlier the Prince had been criticized for performing the ceremony by a leading cancer specialist. Professor Timothy McElwain, of the Royal Marsden, Sutton, Surrey, said he would be giving the seal of approval to unorthodox methods which might raise false hopes in patients.

But the Prince went ahead with his visit to Bristol, watching meditation classes, visiting the kitchens, and seeing counselling and therapy sessions.

Prince Charles told 53-year-old patient Eric Burbridge, of the Fairbank Hotel, Crantock, Newquay, Cornwall, that he looked "extremely well."

Strict

Mr. Burbridge said he had had cancer growths on his back and shoulders and was told there was no hope after several operations.

But he began a strict vegetable diet at the clinic and his growths "exploded" and were rapidly disappearing.

"I feel terrific. I would not be here today but for the treatment I've received," he said.

Among the supporters at yesterday's opening was Dragoon Michael Bentine, a personal friend of the Prince, who said his daughter, Elaine, 41, died from cancer six weeks ago in a Surrey hospital.

His other daughter, Fusty, 33, was now in America where her cancer was being controlled in a similar clinic to the Bristol center.

He said that both women had received personal letters from Prince Charles "mostly about positive thinking."

In his speech, Prince Charles said doctors and healers should work together towards their mutual goal to heal the sick. Alternative methods of treating cancer should not be dismissed as hocus pocus, he said.

Can you imagine the courage it took a world renowned figure such as Prince Charles to step forward and in front of the world take a stand for alternative therapies? Have you any idea what attack he came under just prior to attending the opening of the clinic by all the medical authorities, who tried to stop him. He went through with it, however, and now the doctors are all agreeing that he did the right thing. (If you can't beat them, join them!!!)

NON-TOXIC METABOLIC TREATMENT AND DIET (The New Zealand Guide)

This is also a successful way of overcoming cancers. Vitamins, minerals and enzymes:

Vitamins to take: Vitamin A; Vitamin B1, B2, B17 (Laetrile); Vitamin C; Vitamin E except for cancer of the breast and/or uterus (because of its hormone-like effect).

These are extremely effective in halting and shrinking cancers – especially Vitamins A, E and B17; Vitamin C enhances their efficiency. They should be prescribed by your practitioner in massive doses initially, and then reduced as your cancer shrinks away. N.B. Vitamin B17 (Laetrile) is most effective when intravenously injected.

Minerals to take: To assist the body by promoting the manufacture of enzymes used by the immune system in the destruction of cancer cells. Magnesium; Potassium; Phosphorous; Zinc; Selenium; Calcium; Chromium; (Amounts to be prescribed by your practitioner following blood analysis.)

Enzymes to take: These help to break down the wall of the cancer cells by digesting their muco-protein content. Bromelain; Trypsin; Chymotrypsin; Retenzyme or Wobe Mugos (the latter is more effective but over twice as expense); Pancrex V; (Dosage to be prescribed by your practitioner.)

Typical daily amounts of vitamins and enzymes would

be as follows **for an adult cancer patient. Remember, however, to consult your practitioner, as every patient has individual needs.**

Brewer's Yeast Tablets 3x3 daily are a cheap source of the Vitamin B group and include Chromium, protein and an anti-diabetic factor. If these are taken, no Vitamin B1 need be added.

Vitamin A 25,000 i.u. (1,000 mg).

This is best taken in the form of liquidized carrot juice with a little cold-pressed vegetable oil whisked into it. Taken this way the maximum effect of the Vitamin is made use of by the body to attack the cancer. The Vitamin A tablets tends to be stored in the liver for gradual release and is therefore not so effective.

Vitamin B1 - 10 to 20 mg.

Vitamin B2 - 30 mg.

N.B Vitamins B6, B12 and Folic Acid increase the growth of cancers, so do not take these.

Vitamin C - 2 to 5 grams per day (2,000 to 5,000 mg).

Magnesium Orotate - 1,000 mg per day.

Zinc - 15 mg (but only in cases of zinc deficiency).

Calcium - 1,500 mg.

Selenium - 200 micrograms.

Manganese - 5 to 20 mg.

Jason Winters Red Clover Enzymes.

(Two tablets three times a day **between** meals, i.e. on an **empty** stomach. Start with a much lower dose and gradually increase to this amount.)

Vitamin D - Amygdalin Injections or Tablets.

Although Amygdalin can be intravenously injected, the Cancer Help Center, Bristol, is currently suggesting the following: 15 apricot kernels orally administered three times a day or 250 mg Amygdalin tablets thrice daily over an extended period plus 2 grams of Vitamin C plus 20 to 30 oz. of emulsified carotene (as described on previous page) per day plus enzymes. If large doses of Amygdalin are given intravenously, the products of cyanide detoxification (thiocyanates) gradually accumulate and there is a loss of appetite. The combination of Vitamins C, A and enzymes is necessary for Amygdalin to work satisfactorily.

CARCINOGENS TO AVOID

1. Carcinogens in daily use or commonly occurring:

Tobacco smoke, whether or not you are the smoker. (Especially bad for lung and bladder cancer.)

Coal tar and petrochemical derivatives used in toothpaste, hair oils, lipsticks and cosmetics, perfumes, soaps, deodorants, anti-perspirants and mouth sprays.

Plastics such as cellophane, nylon, Teflon, Dacron, polyethylene, polystyrene, polyvynilchloride, e.g. food containers, kitchen utensils, clothes, carpets, furniture, curtains, bedding, etc.

Fluoride in water supplies.

Fluoride in toothpaste.

Epoxy resins, glues, etc.

Dust of all kinds (including wood dust, leather dust and especially asbestos dust).

Talcum powder or products containing talc.

Carbon tetrachloride (used in cleaning fluids, etc.)

Many factory emissions.

Car, lorry, bus and boat exhausts.

Aerosol sprays.

Food dyes.

Detergents for washing food utensils (they form free radicals from food in the body).

Food preservatives, especially nitrates in bacon, tinned meat, ham, sausage, etc., but also other chemical additives.

Fumes from central heating boilers (oil, coal or gas-fired).

2. Industrial carcinogens:

Tar; Tar gas; Pitch; Asphalt; Creosote; Cooper; Aniline dye; Nickel; Radon (used in building materials); Plastics; Radium; Uranium; X-rays; Mineral oils (including motor oils and greases); Arsenic; Asbestos.

3. Medical carcinogens:

Reserpine (suspect); Chloroform; Liquid paraffin; All mineral oil products; Hormone therapy (including contraceptive pills); Selenium Sulphide (suspect); Methapyrilene (suspect); X-rays (including radioactive dyes and radio isotopes); All coal derivatives; Antibiotics and sulphonomide drugs are strongly suspect (certainly they cause animal cancers); Depo Provera is strongly suspect. It is banned in the U.S.A. (injectable contraceptive); Psoralens (used for treating skin complaints); Aldactone and Flagose cause cancer in animals. These are widely used drugs.

4. Other carcinogens:

Background radiation for A and H Bomb explosions, polluting atmosphere, crops, meat and water; Certain fungi — as in some pickled vegetables — especially aflatoxins; Bracken (contains cocetin); Certain viruses; Radiation from TV sets, clocks and watches, etc.; Radiation from the sun.

5. Carcinogens and potential carcinogens in food and drink:

Dyes (e.g. butter yellow); Preservatives, e.g. Nitrates in bacon, sausages, ham and tinned meat and other preservatives; Chlorine in tap water; Pesticides and their residues; Insecticides; Smoked meats and fish (such food often contains creosote and formaldehyde); Nitrates are formed from nitrates and combine with amines in gut to form nitrosamines. Nitrosamines are cancer inducing; Saccharin (chemical sweetener); Fats heated to high temperatures (above 200°C or 392° F) in preparing food. Frying is therefore NOT RECOMMENDED; Coffee is suspect because, in the roasting, matrol is produced. Decaffeinated coffee also contains matrol; Fluoridated water; Saturated fat (found in dairy produce, meat and meat products, pastry, cakes and puddings, cheese, milk, eggs, fish and chips, and other fried foods).

— 27 —

FACTS THAT YOU SHOULD KNOW ABOUT CANCER RESEARCH

*M*any doctors say that the next big illness to come along within the next ten years will make cancer look insignificant. They say it will take that long for the microwave ovens to really start showing just how dangerous they are.

We have discussed the most necessary thing in the world and that is of course, live food. Today twenty-five percent is dead and worthless.

With any food, it's the enzymes that still live that's so important to our even staying alive. Cooked food on a conventional stove leaves some enzymes alive, but a microwave oven kills all the goodness at once, within the first ten seconds. Everything that you eat from a microwave oven is not only useless, but your body has to work very hard to get rid of it quickly, otherwise you become toxic, and that is the beginning of death. These are facts that are widely known by people in authority, but they will not speak out, for they are frightened to take an unpopular stand on any issue.

The following are also facts that have been published and are quite well known in influential circles but nothing is done for the same reason.

Is it possible that anyone could still believe that nuclear testing and nuclear power plants are as wonderful as some try to tell us?

Cancer and 'The Conqueror': An 'epidemic' from nuclear radiation?

NEW YORK (AP) – Cancer hit an unusually high number of the cast and crew of the movie "The Conqueror", which starred the late John Wayne and which was filmed in 1954 near St. George, Utah, a year after nuclear weapons test upwind in Nevada, People magazine reports.

Of the 220 cast and crew members, the magazine said it was able to contact 150 and that 91 of them had contracted cancer.

Forty-six of those who contracted cancer – including Wayne, co-star Susan Hayward and producer-director Richard Powell died of the disease, the magazine said yesterday.

"With these numbers, this case could qualify as an epidemic," the magazine quoted Dr. Robert C. Pendelton, director of radiological health at the University of Utah, as saying.

"The connection between fallout radiation and cancer in individual cases has been practically impossible to prove conclusively. But in a group this size you'd expect only 30-some cancers to develop. With 91, I think the tie-in to their exposure on the set of 'The Conqueror' would hold up even in court."

A report similar to People's was published in June 1979 in London newspapers but was met with skepticism. A spokesman for the Wayne family said then that he had heard the theory but considered it "absolutely not true."

More than 950 residents and former residents of Utah, Nevada and Arizona have filed $2 billion in claims against the federal government, seeking compensation for damages they say are related to fallout. The first of those cases is scheduled to go to trial next September.

Actress Jeanne Gerson, 76, who also appeared in "The Conqueror", told the magazine that she had hired a lawyer to file a class-action suit against the government and said she hoped others involved in the movie would join her. She said she has undergone surgery for skin and breast cancer.

A House Subcommittee said in August that the now-defunct Atomic Energy Commission "not only disregarded but actually suppressed" all evidence of harmful effects of radiation from atmospheric tests in Nevada.

The magazine also said the disease has struck the children of some of the actors who had accompanied their parents to the filming site in Snow Canyon near St. George, 137 miles downwind from the Yucca Flat weapons test range.

Wayne's son Michael, developed skin cancer in 1975, it said. His brother Patrick underwent surgery 11 years ago from a breast tumor, but it was not malignant. Susan Hayward's son, Tim Barker, had a benign tumor removed from his mouth in 1968, but told the magazine, "I still smoke a pack a day."

Wayne died in June 1979 after suffering cancers of the lung, throat and stomach.

War on Cancer Called "Worthless Sham"
— Press Telegram

Critics label prevention way to end disease

WASHINGTON (AP) – Medical experts told a House Subcommittee Tuesday that the nation's war on cancer is being mismanaged and is nearly worthless.

One of the harshest critics of the National Cancer Institute (NCI) and the National Institute of Health (NIH) was Dr. Irwin D. J. Bross, Director of Biostatistics at the Roswell Park Memorial Institute for Cancer Research in Buffalo, New York.

Bross said much of the money Congress has earmarked for cancer research has been "wasted on scientific boondoggles such as the worthless cancer vaccine program" and other activities he said are pushed by technicians seeking part of the anticancer money.

If half of the time, effort and money for the NCI in the past five years had been put into an effective primary prevention program, "we would at this moment be well on our way to the actual conquest of cancer," he contended.

"The programs for environmental carcinogens are little more than public relations gimmicks — paper tigers designed to reassure the concerned public that something is being done when it isn't," he said.

"This is standard policy in NIH. The program on cigarette health hazards is a farce. It consists of noisy scare campaigns which are counter productive – like most of cancer education," he said.

Bross alleged that federal cancer research money is going to "Laboratory scientists who have no real interest in ... human cancer and who couldn't care less about prevention of human disease."

He charged that NCI funds are largely controlled by the American Cancer Society and said it should be barred from getting any NCI grants for the next four years. In any other part of government, Bross said, it would be a corrupt practice for persons giving out the money and persons getting it to be the same.

The critical analysis was given to a House Government Operations Subcommittee as the director of the National Center for Health Statistics conceded that figures indeed show that there is an increased risk of dying of cancer.

The intergovernmental relations and human resources subcommittee, chaired by Rep. L. H. Fountain, D - N. C., is conducting three days of hearings on the $800 million program NCI is managing.

The director of the statistics center, Mrs. Dorothy P. Rice, said the cancer death rate has risen since 1930 from 100 deaths per 100,000 population to 171 deaths per 100,000 for 1975. Preliminary figures indicate that last year's cancer death rate also rose substantially, she said.

Asked the reasons for the upswing, Mrs. Rice said that most of the increase has been due to the aging of the population. The chances of dying from cancer are highest for older persons. Other causes include cigarette smoking and more exposure to industrial environments, she said.

Dr. Sidney M. Wolfe of Ralph Nader's Public Citizen's health Research Group called the national cancer war a "sham battle."

"NCI, under new leadership, must choose to become the leader in the war to prevent cancer, rather than the banking operation for the largely unsuccessful war to treat it (cancer) after it happens," said Wolfe.

He said the NCI should assume a "new role" in actively overseeing "lethargic" regulatory agencies by publishing an "Annual Report of Potential Cancer Victims."

Wolfe suggested that the NCI issue a public warning to pinpoint the known cancer-causing agents to which millions of Americans are exposed because of "negligence" of agencies charged with regulating hazardous chemicals.

He cited eight agents – including arsenic, benzene, chloroform and estrogens – which he said "are exposing more than 17 million Americans to a serious risk of cancer." Adding two commonly used red dyes "probably increases this total to over 100 million people," he said.

Wolfe and Bross both accused the government of yielding to pressures of profit by emphasizing after-the-fact diagnosis and treatment at the expense of preventative measures during the first five years of the proclaimed "Conquest of Cancer" effort.

Bross has persistently opposed x-ray screening of younger women in the breast cancer program – a procedure that has recently been discontinued for routine use on women under 50.

Bross charged that the screening program and attempts to develop a cancer vaccine were "boondoggle" examples of the "incredibly bad management that has plagued the 'Conquest of Cancer' program."

He urged more "public accountability" by government agencies that "continue to see themselves as the patrons of the medical establishment and not as servants of the public."

This theme has been sounded frequently as more cancer-causing agents have been identified and the death toll has continued to grow.

Fountain said that "in 1957, the same proportion of cancer cases – one in three – was being cured," he had been informed. If that information is correct, he said, "we will want to know why, despite all of the effort and money devoted to cancer research in the past 20 years, the cure rate has remained unchanged."

SPECIAL REPORT FROM THE MIAMI CONVENTION

Thousands came out to see Jason Winters after hearing him on numerous radio shows in the Miami area. The Miami Herald was also very kind to us all.

It was the same old story; many happy old customers, hundreds of new ones and some very disgruntled at finding out from Jason that they had been wasting money on the wrong products.

One nutritionist that was trying to sell a diet book was so upset at Jason's massive following and easy style, he told listeners on a radio show; **Jason Winters is unscientific.** While I, on the other hand have been mentioned in medical books many times. Jason Winters is totally unscientific!! Jason's immediate reply made listeners cheer with delight, as it was so unexpected. "Yes, I am completely 100% unscientific, after all, it was science that sent me home to die. I am as unscientific as love, hope, faith, the Bible, christianity. I am as unscientific as the 1 ½ billion people of the world that use herbs daily, they too have no explanation, only results."

— *28* —

YOUR WEAKNESS & YOUR HERB ACCORDING TO YOUR BIRTHSIGN

THE HERB JUST MEANT FOR YOU

*T*housands of years ago, the Chinese Emperor Sheng Noong compiled a list of 365 herbs and their known uses. He came upon this knowledge from his ancient ancestors who, through trial and error over the centuries, found the true value of each herb.

One almost forgotten piece of information passed down to him, and to almost every ancient tribe from each continent is that people born under certain signs have certain body weaknesses and only certain herbs can help them.

To know the herb that is meant for you can be important. Also, knowing the weakness in you due to your birth sign is proving not only invaluable but remarkably accurate.

Here then is the ancient list of herbs according to the twelve signs of the zodiac.

ARIES

The complaints of Aries are: fevers, problems of the face and head.

ARIES HEALING HERBS ARE: Cayenne, Honeysuckle, Garlic and Blessed Thistle, with Garlic and Honeysuckle being the most important.

TAURUS

The complaints of Taurus are: problems with the neck and throat due to overeating or other excesses, sometimes an emotional problem.

TAURUS HEALING HERBS ARE: Thyme, Tansy Plantain and Silverweed, with Thyme being the most important.

GEMINI

The complaints of Gemini are: bronchial infections, nervousness, pains in the arms and shoulder and incorrect breathing causing brain fevers.

GEMINI HEALING HERBS ARE: Meadowsweet, Skullcap and Flax, with the Skullcap being the most important.

CANCER

The complaints of Cancer are: indigestion, weakness of the chest such as asthma, cancer and stomach troubles.

CANCER HEALING HERBS ARE: Violet, Butterbur and Ground Ivy, with the Violet being the most important.

LEO

The complaints of Leo are: sore eyes, fevers, cramps, palpitations and heart problems.

LEO HEALING HERBS ARE: St. John's Wort, Mistletoe and Eyebright, with St. John's Wort being the most important.

VIRGO

The complaints of Virgo are: all problems of the liver, intestines and solar plexus.

VIRGO HEALING HERBS ARE: Fennel, Marshmallow and Blue Flag, with Fennel being the most important.

LIBRA

The complaints of Libra are: kidneys, stones, pains in the back, bladder and over acidity.

LIBRA HEALING HERBS ARE: Burdock, Pennyroyal, Archangel, with Burdock being the most important.

SCORPIO

The complaints of Scorpio are: problems with the generative organs, piles, catarrh in the bladder, uterine.

SCORPIO HEALING HERBS ARE: Wormwood, Toad Flax, Red Clover, with Wormwood being the most important.

SAGITTARIUS

The complaints of Sagittarius are: goiter, pain in lower limbs, fevers and over exercise, also cancer of the intestines and liver.

SAGITTARIUS HEALING HERBS ARE: Agrimony, Red Clover, Chaparral, and Tribalene, with Tribalene being the most important.

CAPRICORN

The complaints of Capricorn are: corns, warts, skin diseases, ruptures and weakness of the lower limbs.

CAPRICORN HEALING HERBS ARE: Slippery Elm, Shave Grass, Thyme, Comfrey, Shepherds Purse, with Comfrey being the most important.

AQUARIUS

The complaints of Aquarius are: Toxic blood, paralysis, eye problems, Rheumatic Fever.

AQUARIUS HEALING HERBS ARE: Tribalene, Ragwort, Wood Sage, Blue Vervain, with Tribalene being the most important.

PISCES

The complaints of Pisces are: painful feet and toes, gout, ulcers, boils, corns, and blood impurities.

PISCES HEALING HERBS ARE: Yarrow, Cayenne, Tribalene, Ginger, with Yarrow being the most important.

ARE HERBS HYGIENIC?

As most people know, I was drinking an herbal formula every day while recovering from terminal cancer. I continued to drink the formula by the gallon. Its taste wasn't that bad.

After full recovery, I had the privilege of meeting Britain's herbalist expert who really taught me a lot about herbs. It seems that if you are able to go into the country and pick your own herbs, take them home and clean them with fresh water, all is fine. But most people buy their herbs from a store, and this is where the trouble starts because the herbs could have been picked last year, and maybe sat in a warehouse for six months before packaging, then mixed into tea and have sat on a shelf at the store ever since.

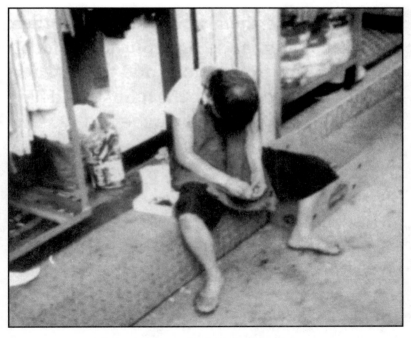

Opium destroys the life of many Asians.

Most of the goodness has gone. It was this that started an investigation on just how to prepare herbs so that the goodness of the herbs remain. We left this problem for our scientists to figure out while I went to Denmark to watch a crop of red clover be cut and gathered by a farmer. My combination of herbs are cleaned and sifted three times, not once like the other companies, then subjected to a special purifying treatment that eliminates everything else but leaves the goodness intact. It is ground up at temperatures below freezing and placed in a capsule or shaker to be spread on food. We have been told by the herb people in California that this system is the cleanest and safest way to prepare herbs and other large companies have already started offering to purchase the system so that they can present a better product also.

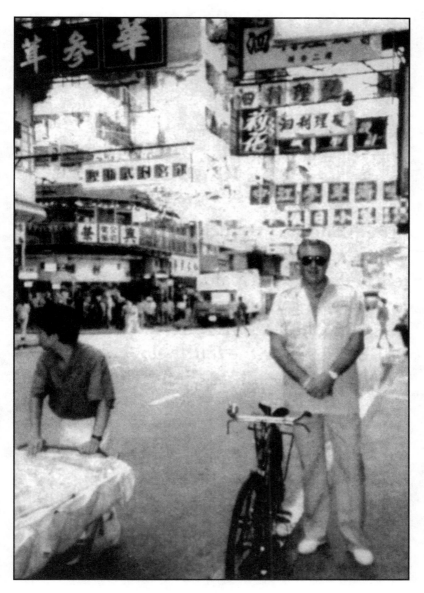

The search for herbs in China.

THE REASON

*T*he London taxi driver dropped me off outside a four-story terrace house that had seen better days. I paid him and he quickly drove off. The sign on the door read "SCIENTIFIC RESEARCH FOR THE PREVENTION OF DISEASE." It was on the fourth floor and with no elevator, it was quite a climb. The office was small, and was equipped with a very old lady and a very new computer. I had no appointment, and had decided to give my name as Mr. Goodman, just in case they had heard of me. I wanted to test them fully.

Mrs. Higgins didn't even look at me as she started her running commentary which seemed to bore even her. "We at the center give each person certain forms containing 152 questions. You must answer them absolutely truthfully or its a waste of our time and yours. When you have completed the questionnaires, you must send it back to this office with a cheque in the amount of twenty pounds.

We put your answers into the computer, and they are

analyzed. In due time you will receive a complete summary of the illnesses you are prone to, the ones you must watch out for. The computer will know this from the kind of stress you have been subjected to, the emotional side and also the type of childhood that you have had. Thank you and goodbye Mr. Goodman!"

I found myself out on the street within five minutes of my arrival, and I had not had the chance to ask even one of the thousand questions that I had planned to. To make matters worse, I had to walk about two miles before I could hail a cab. While I walked I found I kept muttering to myself, "that woman was enough to give anyone stress, talk about computers taking over," and on and on I complained.

Once back at the Grosvenor House Hotel I read the forms, which were both difficult yet simple. Simple questions, but they raked up a lot of very unhappy memories for me. It took me over five hours to answer the 152 questions honestly, and the next morning I sent the forms back to Mrs. Higgins along with the cheque. None of the questions were about illness or about previous health problems.

In three weeks, the dreaded report came. It was exactly as follows:

REPORT 6303:JASON GOODMAN (WINTERS) LYNDON FILE

Born as the third child to a very unhappy couple. Father asthmatic, mother neurotic, having many affairs. Subject was the result of one such union with a neighbor. Mother would tell her friends how hard she had tried to terminate the pregnancy, and this in front of the child. Mother would call the subject a freak because he was well over six feet tall at fourteen years of age.

Both the subject's sisters had great animosity towards subject, with no affection whatsoever. Mother told subject constantly that he was not as good as the others. He was also expected to fail. Sisters also found it impossible to give love and affection.

Subject grew up in an atmosphere of selfishness, bitterness and hatred, with no love, compassion or even interest for his future.

Subject had a most unhappy childhood, and is typical of a future cancer victim. Out of the six thousand five hundred cases studied so far, an astounding 78% had similar unhappy backgrounds and most developed cancer.

Subject should be wary of nose, throat, tongue, and mouth problems, including cancer.

———————————

I had already suffered terminal cancer of the tongue, jaw bone, tonsils and mouth, but they did not know that. I thought that this was remarkable.

I could not help remembering that when I did come down with terminal cancer, my sister was two blocks away, but she would not come to see me. She has also never congratulated me regarding beating cancer, and has chosen never to mention my top-selling book, or the work we are doing world wide. A close source has said that she would have rather I had died than become successful.

Because of this, may I urge all parents to please give openly of their love. Don't be afraid to show affection, hug your kids regularly. If parents only realized the importance of raising children, of telling them that they are good, nice, sweet, and that you love them, they would do it all the time.

Mothers, possibly you have a chance to turn a child into a great person, a world leader, or just another great parent. Give them love today and the world will be in good hands tomorrow.

— 30 —

PROBLEMS ARE
ILLUSIONS

*T*he old man frightened me because he was so old and was obviously dying. I tried to smile but he saw the tears in my eyes. "Do not cry for me my son, for even in one million years we will both still be in existence."

We worry so much about nothing that we make ourselves sick. When we are not worrying, we worry about why we are not worrying. But it's as all religions tell us, it is all an illusion.

For instance, you are not short of money, just short of ideas, because money rushes to ideas.

You are not unemployed, you are just trained for the wrong job.

You don't disagree with your spouse, you just don't know how to communicate.

You are not terminal, you just don't know about eternal life.

You must get up and get going, for not even GOD can steer a parked car.

It is said that a lifetime of tragedy and sorrow is forgotten in a second, once you gaze on the face of Jesus.

All you have to do is furnish the sinner, HE will furnish the saviour. Even the blind beggar sitting on the road to Jericho knew the secret and was healed, so don't despair, your faith will set you free.

> Shackled with a heavy burden
> full of sin and shame
> and suddenly HE touched me
> and I will never be the same.

PORTRAIT OF CHRIST

*It shows in your face: A description of Jesus
from the Roman Archives.*

*A*bout 2,000 years ago, a Roman named Publius Lentulus wrote a report to his emperor, Tiberius, and included the following description of the man known as Jesus Christ: "A tall, well proportioned man, his hair is the color of new wine ... curled as it falls to (his shoulders). Upon the forehead, it parts in two. His forehead is flat and fair, his face without blemish or defect and adorned with a graceful expression. His nose and mouth are very well proportioned; his beard thick and the color of his hair, red gold. His eyes are gray and extremely lively. He is the handsomest man in the world."

— The report is kept in the Archives in Rome.

If you wish to be placed on the Jason Winters mailing list, and to receive free copies of the "NEW AGE ADVISOR" which tells of Jason's travels, progress and discoveries, please send your name and address to:

VINTON PUBLISHING
PO BOX 94075
LAS VEGAS, NEVADA 89197

There is no charge for this service.

On December 7th, 1984, Jason Winters was summoned to attend the World Health Conference in Madrid, Spain. With over two thousand specialists attending, Jason Winters was presented with the "Medal of Honor" by Sir Henk Oswald of Holland. He was also appointed Laureate of Belgium, The Netherlands and South Africa. This award originated with King Albert I of Belgium. In a later speech in London which caused great applause, Prince Obazee of Nigeria stated that Sir Jason Winters has "done more for humanity than any other single individual alive today."

SUMMATION AND BELIEFS

I do not believe that the herbs mentioned in this book cure any illnesses or disease. I think that they do one thing, and that is to purify the blood. Once this is done then the immune system can start to work to heal your own body. Your body actually heals itself.

God in His wisdom put a special herb on each continent to do just one thing, purify a persons blood. Knowing full well that when this was done a persons body would heal itself. In biblical times, before fluoride in the water, polluted air, processed food, any one of these herbs would have worked, but not today. Our blood is so toxic that it takes the combined efforts of the three herbs from the three continents to really work well. This is what the author did by accident many years ago.

There is no person or company associated with Jason Winters that believes any other than the above.

Every religion since the beginning of time emphasizes the importance of the blood. That's what I really meant by "the blood of Christ," the saying "life is in the blood" and "purify your blood with herbs and all things fall away." We have an immune system, all we need to do is to help it out a little.

It's no accident that the Aborigines, Africans, Indians, Arabs, Chinese, Tibetans all purify their blood on a daily basis. We in North America do not, and our sickness and death rate is the highest it has ever been.

ONE REASON WHY

A Tibetan wakes in the morning, stretches, yawns, looks out at the sun and smiles. He thanks God that he is alive, and fully expects a long happy life and a very good day, and so that's what he gets.

We in the west wake up and turn on television. A top star is telling us that if we get sick at our age it's going to wipe us out financially. Our medical coverage just isn't enough, we must pay for more. We turn the channel in disgust to hear a man shouting "buy your burial plot today, don't leave it to your children!!" One more channel change brings on a doctor telling us to "look for lumps in the breasts each day, check for moles that are changing, rush to your doctor, check your blood pressure at the supermarket. Thoroughly depressed we pour white sugar and cream all over our crispy crunchy cereal, wash it down with three cups of black coffee, light up a cigarette and cough and wheeze all the way to the office where we must perform well every day for our boss, or he will hire someone younger to take our place for less money. It doesn't matter how well you did last year or even last week, you must perform well today or else!

Is this really what God wanted for you, His perfect creation? No, of course not, but there is a way out, as millions have found, for that one little sentence can change your life, yes **"life is in the blood."**